Horses, Heifers and Hairy Pigs

Horses, Heifers and Hairy Pigs

THE LIFE OF A
YORKSHIRE VET

JULIAN NORTON

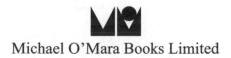

Michael O'Mara Books Limited

First published in Great Britain in 2016 by
Michael O'Mara Books Limited
9 Lion Yard
Tremadoc Road
London SW4 7NQ

A CIP catalogue record for this book is available from the British Library.

Papers used by Michael O'Mara Books Limited are natural, recyclable products made
from wood grown in sustainable forests. The manufacturing processes conform to the
environmental regulations of the country of origin.

ISBN: 978-1-78243-683-6 in hardback print format
ISBN: 978-1-78243-684-3 in ebook format

1 2 3 4 5 6 7 8 9 10

www.mombooks.com

Typeset by Jade Wheaton

Printed and bound by CPI Group (UK) Ltd, Croydon, CR0 4YY

CONTENTS

Dedicated to the memory of Dave Payne,
great friend, superb climber, typical Yorkshireman.
Died on the Matterhorn, August 1993

*

And for Anne: thank you for putting up with me,
for skilfully fine-tuning my stories and for not cutting
out too many of my words

Foreword by Jim Wight

My father and I had almost finished a busy evening surgery at the veterinary practice of Sinclair and Wight in Thirsk. There was just one client left to see; he was sitting patiently and, on his knee, there was a large cardboard box with holes in. Rustling noises emanated from within the box.

'I can tell you two things about whatever is inside that box,' said my father with a wry smile. 'It'll be fast ... and it'll bite. You can deal with it!'

'Thanks, Dad!'

As a practising veterinary surgeon with almost fifty years' experience of working in general practice, my father, Alf Wight, had observed tremendous changes within his profession. Writing as James Herriot, he had brilliantly documented the ever-evolving face of the veterinary profession. He was a traditional vet – domestic farm animals, cats and dogs – and he faced, reluctantly, having to turn his hand to the 'exotic' species, for example rabbits, hamsters, gerbils, tortoises and snakes. He would have been amazed to observe the work of the vets at the Skeldale Veterinary Centre – the modern, relocated veterinary practice in Thirsk – as they tackle the many and varied ailments of so many different species. Their work has captured the interest of viewers nationwide as they watch *The Yorkshire Vet* television series on Channel 5. This programme has proved extremely popular, and just like James Herriot decades ago, they are a credit to their profession, accurately depicting the busy life of today's practising veterinarians.

The profession has endured a barrage of criticism over recent years, with the accusation of vets charging extortionate fees a prime example. It should be remembered that the modern veterinary practice, in satisfying an ever more demanding public, faces huge overheads in providing a comprehensive, up-to-date and first-class service to their clients. This they largely do, and while watching *The Yorkshire Vet* there is little indication of any financial gain being the prime motivation. Just as James Herriot depicted his profession as the caring one, this television series projects a similar image. Many things have changed since James Herriot's heyday, but in this respect, not much has altered.

My father often said that his time in veterinary practice was 'harder but more fun'. It was certainly physically harder, but in contrast to his day, the modern vet has to deal with an endless onslaught of rules and regulations, with the threat of litigation lurking round every corner. Despite this, the vets and staff at Skeldale maintain an upbeat and humorous approach to their work, something that my father would have applauded. He always maintained that laughter was an essential ingredient of every veterinary surgeon's day, and there was plenty of humour in his days as a vet, something that is more than adequately recorded in his bestselling books.

Julian, with whom I worked only very briefly, as I was retiring while he was beginning his time in Thirsk, mentions in his book how he too, over a comparatively short period of twenty years or so, has noticed the great changes in the work of the veterinary surgeon. When I began my time as a vet in Thirsk in 1967, the practice of Sinclair and Wight had between ninety and one hundred dairy farms to visit; now the Skeldale Veterinary Centre has only two or three. The country vet's life was one of visiting countless small family farms, a time when the vet was almost a member of the family. They were days when a man milking twenty cows could make a decent living; at the time of writing this foreword, a dairy farmer milking ten times that number is struggling to make ends meet.

Most of our small farms have disappeared, many of them absorbed into much larger enterprises. Family-run veterinary practices have faced similar challenges, with large organizations swallowing up the smaller businesses. I believe it is refreshing to see local practices, like the one here in Thirsk, doing so well and providing an excellent twenty-four-hour, seven days a week, service in the face of so many big takeovers in our profession.

The Yorkshire Vet series has proved a great success, partly due to the honest and dedicated treatment of the patients, as displayed on the television screen. This is veterinary practice as it really is, and despite the many changes that have occurred since my time as a vet, some things have not changed, and I relive quite a few memories while watching the programme.

In this book, Julian gives a realistic insight into life behind the scenes at Skeldale Veterinary Centre, a turbulent life of triumphs mixed with disappointments. James Herriot said many times that he felt he was the greatest vet on earth one minute, only to feel a total idiot the next. This is adequately illustrated in Julian's book and, as the reader will realize, it has done nothing to dampen his enthusiasm. His love for his profession is very clear; the elation following a successful case, his despair when things do not go to plan, together with his outspoken views on such important topics as tuberculosis and foot and mouth disease.

Shortly following my father's death, a statement from the British Veterinary Association read, 'James Herriot's scientific and technical approach to his cases may well be outdated, but his caring and compassionate approach to both patient and customer is most definitely not'. The vets and staff at Skeldale Veterinary Centre are carrying forward that James Herriot tradition of compassion and care into the modern age. Long may this continue.

Jim Wight, BVMS, MRCVS, author of *The Real James Herriot*

Introduction

The pregnant cow had no intention of going into the cattle crush inside the barn. She wasn't used to being handled by humans, having spent most of her life out on the moor, and we had been struggling to catch her for half an hour. Eventually we managed to lasso her and get a halter on, but she still stubbornly refused to go in to the rusty old crush, so we had to make do with just tying her to it, via the halter. The poor girl was giving birth, but her calf was enormous. There was no way it could be born without a caesarean section.

It was hard to see what I was doing in the gloomy light of the barn, but apart from the well-aimed and unpredictable kicks from my patient, the operation was going smoothly. The calf was sturdy and full of vigour, and was soon rolling around in the straw looking for its mother. Then, just as I was about to start suturing everything back together, disaster struck.

The cow jumped in the air. Both the cattle crush and the halter were old and worn out, and the halter quickly gave way. The cow, unaccustomed to being in a barn, raised her head, opened her eyes wide and charged, looking either for revenge, her calf, or a means of escape. There was a large open doorway in the barn, and this offered a clear route to the moorland beyond. If she chose escape, she would be loose on the moors with her uterus dangling from the large hole in her left flank, through which her calf had been delivered. This would be a catastrophe. The farmer and I could only stand and watch, as the cow chose her fate. She stopped her charge and looked out at the moorland, then turned back to look at her calf. Thankfully, her maternal instincts were strong. As she settled with her baby, we managed to fasten her up again so I could suture her uterus and her flank and finish the operation.

I drove back home that evening as the sun was setting, feeling very lucky. It was a great story, and reminded me of a conversation I'd had with my English teacher, Mr Clough, many years before.

'Well, Julian,' he had implored, 'if you are determined to become a vet, will you promise me one thing – you will, at least, write about being one?'

'I'll see what I can do, sir,' I assured him. Inwardly, I suspected that this was highly unlikely. I had yet to sit my GCSE examinations and could only dream of a place at veterinary school. The path to becoming a veterinary surgeon was beset by many hurdles, and it seemed ludicrous to imagine that I could become both a vet and an author.

But twenty-eight years later, hurdles negotiated, here I was, a veterinary surgeon, working in a wonderful mixed practice in my beloved North Yorkshire. It was, in fact, the practice where the most famous vet of them all, James Herriot, spent his working life, and from where he penned the iconic books that inspired a generation of veterinary surgeons. I thought myself pretty fortunate. Life was good, but very hectic. Work was tough and busy, I was training to compete for the GB triathlon team, had two very sporty boys, and a wife who was also a vet and also very busy. We had many balls to keep in the air. After being called out during one night at 2 a.m., 4 a.m. and 6 a.m., to replace uterine prolapses in three different cows (a heavy and dirty job), I remember thinking that I could not possibly fit anything else into my life.

So, when the practice was approached, by Daisybeck Studios, about the possibility of making a television series called *The Yorkshire Vet*, we all had mixed feelings. It would be a lot of extra work for everyone and we would be putting the practice, our clients and ourselves on public display. But I thought it could be a fun and different way of approaching the summer's work. It would be a good advert for our modern but traditional mixed practice, and our links with James Herriot could not be overlooked. So we agreed to be filmed over the summer of 2015, with enthusiasm from some of us, and hesitation from others.

What followed was one of the most challenging periods of my professional life. Being filmed felt like doing two jobs at once, and I had thought doing just one was pretty hard. However, the series proved to be more popular than any of us would have dreamt, and soon the cameras were back, to start filming for a second series. Minor (very minor) celebrity status followed. I was asked to open a shop selling Christmas trees, I had a 'selfie' taken with the fishmonger in the market square and modelled shirts for a local clothes retailer. I was even recognized as I queued at the check-in desk at the airport and my eldest son temporarily thought I was a cool dad, rather than an embarrassing one. Although I was still just doing what I had always done, things had definitely changed and soon the chance arose to write a book, so I was able to follow the advice of my English teacher at last.

'It will be easy,' the publicity people said, 'we will just send a ghost writer. You cannot possibly work, film for a second series *and* write you own book' (and also train for the Patrouille des Glaciers, a ski mountaineering race through the highest mountains in Switzerland, for which my team and I had just got a much-coveted place). But then, I thought, it wouldn't be my own book. My wife, Anne, agreed to help me. She had some experience writing for newspapers, so we decided upon a strategy. I wrote, and Anne bent and battered it into shape.

James Herriot brought veterinary medicine and Thirsk to the attention of the world. I hope he would recognize and enjoy my version of both. And Mr Clough, I have saved a copy for you!

1

Hard Work and Determination

It seems to me, that the way life develops is a mixture of fate, luck, hard work, determination and making the most of the opportunities that come your way. I don't know whether it is simply good luck that these opportunities appear, or whether it is one's ability to make the most of them. However, as I sit in the dark kitchen of our house, having woken up at 5 a.m. to start writing this book, in the same street that Alf Wight, who wrote under the name of James Herriot, the world's most famous veterinary surgeon, lived for much of his working life, the feeling of destiny is strong. The story of how I became a vet and how I ended up at Skeldale Veterinary Centre in Thirsk, on the edge of the North York Moors, feels similarly preordained.

I did not come from a farming background, or even a rural one, as many aspiring veterinary surgeons did at that time. Far from it, in fact. I was born and brought up in the coalmining town of Castleford, in industrial West Yorkshire. If my choice of career was determined by my birthplace alone, then I should have become a rugby league player, as Wheldon Lane, where Castleford Rugby League team played, was only a short walk from our house. But, while I loved watching the game, I had no talent whatsoever for playing it. I did, however, have plenty of exposure to animals from a young age, because my grandfather kept a smallholding where he reared pigs and turkeys and he also ran a small boarding kennel. My grandparents lived just ten houses up the street from us, so even when I was very young, I would take myself up there at every spare opportunity to help out. They also bred Bedlington terriers. Nowadays, these dogs are neatly trimmed and take pride of place in the show ring, but back then they were tough dogs for rabbiting and catching the rats that were attracted to the pigs and their food at the bottom of the garden. I loved these dogs and I can still remember being able to stand next to Judy the Bedlington terrier when I was small. I could rest my face against her soft, woolly fur and breathe in that unmistakable smell of dog that I now encounter on a nearly daily basis.

My mother was a pharmacist and worked in several of the independent chemist shops in Castleford. I would sometimes have to go along after school to wait for the end of her shift in the dispensary. I watched her counting tablets and measuring out medicines in her clinically clean white coat. Again, I can remember the smell – a mixture of hospitals and chemistry labs – and I was captivated by the process of dispensing these medicines, all for the purpose of treating illness in the patients for whom they were prescribed. So, even at this early age, some seeds were set in my mind for a future career, which must surely involve animals and medicine. And so, as I got older and began to do well at school, particularly in the sciences (my father was a chemistry teacher, so I had no excuses), I began to consider a career as a veterinary surgeon. Undoubtedly, the TV series *All Creatures Great and Small*, based upon Alf Wight's books, which starred Christopher Timothy as James Herriot and Robert Hardy as Siegfried Farnon, was instrumental in my decision. It was on television at about six o'clock on a Sunday evening, and was regular viewing for the whole family.

At this time, I was also an enthusiastic runner. Most of my weekends were taken up with cross country or fell races all over Yorkshire, often in the Dales or the Moors. I loved it, and it became my passion to head to the hills at every opportunity. It did not bother me one bit if the weather was cold, raining, windy or snowing, just as long as I could get outside, into the fresh air and the spectacular scenery for which I was developing an affinity. As it transpired, it was an affinity that would only get stronger. The combination of my love of animals and an overpowering passion for the outdoors made a career in veterinary medicine the obvious choice. Thinking back, I guess the olfactory stimuli of pigs, Bedlington terriers, pharmacies and fresh air was the perfect combination to set me on this path.

I have a photograph of me, as a reticent thirteen-year-old, standing under an archway at Pembroke College, Cambridge. I am wearing one of those plastic macs that nobody wears any more, which afford limited protection from the rain and zero protection from the cold. I loved that mac, though, because it was my running top, and my first piece of proper sporting clothing. Its back was invariably splattered in mud, which left indelible marks, but I used to wear it everywhere. Anyway, I came to be posing for a photo under this archway because my family had taken a day trip to visit Cambridge, one Easter holiday. Parking in Cambridge was (and still is) very difficult but my father had found a parking spot on Trumpington

Street and, as we embarked on our tour around the town, Pembroke College was the first one we visited.

Cambridge is a wonderful place, especially at Easter because the college grounds are bursting with spring flowers, and after walking under that archway there was the most beautifully peaceful courtyard, crammed full of crocuses and daffodils. I immediately set my heart on coming to this place for my university career. As there were only six universities at that time that offered veterinary medicine, I actually didn't have too much choice over which one I applied to, but within Cambridge, I could apply to any one of about twenty-five colleges. However, there was no question in my mind that Pembroke was the place for me, and so it turned out ...

A-levels came and went. As I checked my results on the window at school in the summer of 1990, with a face as fat as a hamster, having just had my wisdom teeth removed, I knew that hard work and determination, luck and fate had given me the opportunity that I wanted.

And so I began my six-year stint at Cambridge to learn how to become a veterinary surgeon. It was an amazing time. Everything was vibrant, full of colour, fun, humour and vitality, and everyone there was larger than life. It was a place full of opportunity, equality and enthusiasm, drive and passion, and it was a wonderful place to spend six years. I would urge any aspiring schoolchild to aim for Cambridge, if they want to be immersed in the heady atmosphere of academia and talent, where anything seems possible and you are judged only upon your merits.

My first few days at Pembroke were spent getting used to the college and its traditions, many of which had probably remained unchanged during its 600-year history. Everything was new to me, a youngster from a Yorkshire mining town, but I quickly felt at home and settled into its peculiar ways. One of our first jobs on arrival was to acquire a gown. A gown was required for formal occasions, and the first of these was the matriculation ceremony, which was a grand affair held on our first weekend. The gown would see us through our undergraduate careers. A few people would buy one, but the sensible approach was to 'borrow' one from the college for three years, in return for a donation to the charity of choice for that year. I was instructed to go into a cloakroom to pick one. There, I found a row of short, black gowns, hanging on pegs. They were all of a similar size, except one, at the end, which had long tassles and extended to the floor. Without thinking, or really knowing what I needed, I immediately picked this one, paid my money and took it back to my room. Little did I know that this was a graduate gown, reserved for students who already had a degree, unlike the short, undergraduate gowns, which all my contemporaries had. I attended every formal occasion wearing this incorrect and completely inappropriate gown. I had many comments – 'Why is your gown so long?' – but I was never reprimanded, simply looked upon with gentle amusement.

My next major error in etiquette and decorum came the very next day. I had resolved to attend evensong at the chapel. This was not particularly because of a strong religious conviction, but more to see what it was all about. The chapel was designed and built by Sir Christopher Wren, the same chap who built St Paul's Cathedral. It was an impressive building and I thought it appropriate to experience it as soon as I could. Evensong started at 6.30 p.m. and finished at 7.15 so most people would eat at formal hall afterwards. However, I decided to opt for the basic option of normal hall at six o'clock, which meant I was running late. As I rushed to the chapel, the congregation was already seated. The choir was just about to begin its procession, followed by the Dean and the Master of the college. As the organ fell silent, to announce the arrival of the important guests, I burst in. This would have been dramatic enough, but the scenario was made worse by the presence of a six-inch step and an excessively long gown. The step was almost invisible since it was very dark. Needless to say, I tripped over the step, and the gown, and made a most spectacular and ridiculous entrance. I picked myself up, straightened my long robes, and looked for a seat. It was very full, being the first evensong of the term, but I spotted an empty seat at the end of a row, opposite the choir stalls. It looked ideal, and was very comfortable with a big cushion. It even had a special place to rest my hymnbook. I settled down, trying to look inconspicuous. Sadly, this was not to be. The choir came in, followed by the Master, who took his place directly opposite me, in an identical seat. Then came the Dean, who looked bemused and then squeezed himself in with the rest of the congregation. It slowly dawned on me that I was sitting in his seat, the most important seat in this historic chapel. No wonder it was so comfy.

After these first few days, settling into our individual colleges, it was time to begin the serious business of learning to be a vet. I nervously made my way to the anatomy department, where I met, for the first time, the fellow veterinary students with whom I would spend the next six happy years, and with whom I would forge some life-long friendships. Our very first task was to be photographed for identification purposes, to allow us entry to the anatomy building. This was necessary because we shared the building with the medics.

While we dissected greyhounds, the medics didn't, so there was attendant security. The photos were pinned to the notice board for all to see. It was a good way of checking people's names, especially when you realized, slightly too many weeks after being introduced, that you couldn't remember someone's name at all. One face sprung out immediately. It was that of a bloke sporting an eighteen-year-old's moustache. He stood out like a sore thumb. That sort of facial furniture was not common or popular in the early 1990s, unless you were co-pilot to Tom Cruise in *Top Gun*. What I couldn't know, though, was that six years later I would be sharing a house and working with this guy, as a friend and colleague at Skeldale Veterinary Centre in Thirsk.

Pembroke College was a great place to be a vet student, mainly because it was right next to the Downing Site, where first year teaching took place. This was good for me, because I could walk to lectures rather than risk life and limb cycling through the rush-hour traffic in the middle of Cambridge. It also meant I could stay in bed for an extra ten minutes in the morning. Some days would start at 5 a.m. with a trip to the river for rowing, and every day would end at 1 a.m. in someone's room after an evening in the college bar, so any opportunity for extra sleep was to be grabbed with both hands.

Equally, it was a bad place to be a vet student, because unlike most of the colleges, which would have anything from two to eight vets, Pembroke rarely took veterinary students at all and, if they did, it was only in ones or twos. There were no vets in either of the two years above me and, as I was the only vet in my year at Pembroke, I was actually the only one in the college. However, I was one of four Julians in the year, so I quickly became known as 'Julian the Vet'. This nickname was soon abbreviated to 'the Vet' and that was my name for the next three years. Obviously it disappeared once I moved up to the vet school for my last three years of clinical training, because there I was one of about sixty others!

Terms only lasted eight weeks and, during this time, every moment was crammed with lectures, dissection, laboratory sessions, supervisions (the Cambridge term for tutorials), sport, drinking and all the other things that happen at university. It was a magical place and stimulating on so many levels. As I was situated so close to lectures, I had no need for a bike, unlike nearly everyone else at Cambridge (although my friend Cindy didn't have a bike because she couldn't ride one). I could walk or run everywhere I needed to go and I think this gave me more time to appreciate the city. Walking to the little supermarket in the middle of town took me right past the laboratory where Watson and Crick discovered DNA. It was humbling to be studying at such a famous and illustrious establishment. I can remember one autumn evening walking back to college as the sun was setting orange. Someone was practising the flute with the window open. The whole of New Court was filled with beautiful music that sounded like an open-air concert. Everybody did things well at Cambridge.

The first three years of the veterinary course were referred to as pre-clinical. This was the theoretical bit before you got your hands on real animals. Nowadays the courses are more integrated but back then, many of the veterinary students were somewhat frustrated by the lack of animal contact. The science was great, and I relished its academic challenges. But it was during the last three years that we really grew into actual vets. At the beginning of the fourth year, veterinary students moved out of town, to the School of Veterinary

Medicine on Madingley Road, and many of us left our rooms in college and found houses to rent. I was lucky to get a room in a lovely house in the village of Newnham. I shared the house with two medics, who were studying at Addenbrooke's Hospital, and two other vets – Siân and Cath, who are both still great friends. Siân now lives and works just 10 miles away from Thirsk and is a good friend of my wife, Anne. Cath is one of the very few of us from the class of 1996 who is still working in mixed practice, working with all species from cattle to cats. There is a growing tendency in the profession to specialize in just a narrow field.

During these last three years we spent all our time at Madingley Road. We were taught in small 'clinical groups' of six or seven students. We had to choose these groups ourselves, so there was much discussion and debate, as we knew we would have to spend almost every waking hour for the next three years in one another's company. I can't quite remember how my clinical group arose, but this time was amongst the happiest of my whole life, due largely to the good-natured, carefree, but diligent atmosphere that pervaded my group.

My closest friend in the group was Ben. We had been firm friends since the first year, as we sparred with one another to woo the attractive girls in our year. We usually consoled ourselves in mutual failure in this field. Cath, my housemate, was also in our group. She had a gentle manner with animals and her quiet patience was inspiring to us all. There was also Jenny, with whom I had spent two pre-clinical years dissecting a formalin-pickled greyhound in anatomy classes. She was hilarious and wore a permanent smile. Only once did I see her gloomy. This was on the occasion we had been dispatched to disbud calves. This is the process whereby the small, developing horns of young cattle are removed – a good job to send vet students on. We had to work our way through them in batches, injecting local anaesthetic around the base of each horn. We then had to burn out the little rubbery nobble of horn bud, using a red-hot burner. This was completely painless to the little calf because the area was numbed by the anaesthetic, but we still had to be careful. I know one vet who burned down a whole barn when his disbudding iron got knocked out of his hand. There was no such drama this time, but Jenny lost control of the red-hot iron and plunged it straight into my face as I held the calf for her. The circular end of the iron, about the size of a ten-pence piece, hit me right on the upper lip and left a deep red circular burn, rendering me unable to smile or laugh for about a week. Jenny was mortified and extremely apologetic. For me it was a painful inconvenience, mainly because we did a lot of smiling and laughing at that time.

The final member of our group was Claire. I did not know her particularly well at the outset – she was a good friend of Ben's – but by the end of our clinical years we were very close. She was keen on equine work and always felt somewhat out of her depth with farm animals. On one particular day, Claire had been doing early morning inspections of her cases, one of which was a young calf, about three months old. It had been poorly with abdominal pain and weight loss and Claire had examined it thoroughly at 7.30 that morning. At 8 a.m., we had 'rounds' where we would present our hospitalized cases to our fellow students and tutors, discuss their progress and plan their treatment. Claire stood confidently in front of the calf pen, describing how the poor calf was a little bit brighter this morning, had suckled some milk, and had a normal temperature and heart rate. It was still recumbent, she said, but making some progress. Dr Jackson, one of our favourite tutors, stood by, wisely nodding his head. He waited patiently for Claire to finish her soliloquy, and then quietly and politely as ever, simply said, 'Thank you, Claire. But the calf is actually dead.' The poor animal had expired in the minutes between her examination and the start of hospital rounds. I can still picture the redness of Claire's embarrassed face to this day.

Dr Jackson was a popular clinician at the vet school. He was an elderly gentleman, hugely experienced and the epitome of polite calmness. He had the utmost respect for the animals he treated. He never lost his temper and was an inspirational teacher to us all. In winter he always wore a cap and overalls, which made him look exactly like the driver of a steam train.

His finest hour, though, was the final Friday afternoon of the large animal rotation. Our clinical years were divided up into blocks called 'rotations', each lasting two weeks. We would concentrate on specific subjects and Dr Jackson was in charge of the 'large animal, reproduction and obstetrics' rotation. This was timetabled for the demonstration of semen collection in the dog, which was part of our reproduction and obstetrics course, which Dr Jackson also taught. Stories of this lesson were fabled at the vet school, so we all knew what sort of spectacle to expect. So did the large black Labrador who was the subject of the demonstration. Friday afternoons were his favourite part of the week. He leapt out of his kennel with the enthusiasm of a thousand men and, without hesitation, jumped straight onto the examination table. I now know that it is extremely unusual for a dog to jump, voluntarily, onto the table of a veterinary surgery, but Bruno knew what was in store for him on a Friday afternoon. The main challenge was for a group of twelve students (we attended this demonstration with a second clinical group) to remain calm and contain the rising swell of giggles. Veterinary students had even been known to stab themselves in the back of the hand with their scissors, or pinch themselves with artery forceps to curb the impending and uncontrollable hysterics. We just about managed to contain ourselves during the demonstration of the semen sample collection, despite the hilarious grin on the dog's face and the soothing and encouraging words of our tutor. However, his final comment, when he was looking for a volunteer to keep the test tube containing the sample at the correct temperature for analysis, was just too much for most of us: 'Now then, who's got nice warm hands?'

We worked hard and played hard during those years, and it wasn't long before our skills were honed. Term times were intense, and during the university holidays, particularly over our last three years, we were required to 'see practice' at veterinary surgeries to gain experience. This was a crucial part of our training and I quickly realized that spending as much time as possible with veterinary surgeons, good ones, was the way to learn the most.

Seeing practice was fantastic because it meant that I could get back to Yorkshire, the hills and the outdoors. I spent most of my holidays at practices in Wetherby, Skipton and York, as well as further afield in the north of Scotland. This was a great time and I set about trying to ensure that I had seen every procedure at least once and that I had actually done as many as I could. It was an opportunity to get your hands dirty and hopefully not make too many mistakes. Cleaning kennels, washing down lambing pens and cleaning calving jacks were all part of a veterinary student's remit. On one occasion I was dispatched to refill the bottles of antiseptic in the practice's lambing shed. I searched to see which of the large brown bottles I should use. The brown liquid in brown bottles all looked the same to me and I refilled one bottle with what appeared to be the right stuff, thinking nothing more of it until the following day. As I was heading out to help one of the vets with a blood test on a beef suckler herd, I heard a commotion in the lambing shed. A furious vet burst out with a red face and dark brown stained arms. I had topped up the bottle of hand antiseptic with Wellington boot disinfectant! I quickly grabbed the blood sampling tubes and hopped in the car. The mixture of enthusiasm and naïvity, I was realizing, could be a hazard.

Despite these occasional mishaps, my student path was progressing nicely and I collected a handful of prizes during my final year. It was time to look for a job …

Directly after graduation I had arranged to work for a few weeks as a locum in a practice in Thurso in Scotland, where I had spent some time as a student, but my first actual job was to be in Thirsk and this, again, came largely by good fortune. My girlfriend (now wife) Anne was in the year above me at vet school and was already working by the time I was looking for a job. Her close friend from Cambridge, David Sutton, was working in the practice at Thirsk. David is an amazing chap, another of those people who is passionate about his job and life in general. He had been in London acting as veterinary advisor to a children's television programme, and called in to visit me at Cambridge on his journey back to North Yorkshire. He mentioned that there might be a job coming up in Thirsk. I pricked up my ears. This was a mixed practice job – just what I wanted – and it was in North Yorkshire – exactly what I was looking for – so I arranged to call in for an interview.

I was travelling up north the following weekend to organize a stag weekend in the Peak District for my friend Pete, so it fitted in fairly well. I squeezed into my little red Mini Metro and headed up the A1. The Metro was one of those cars that was red when it left the factory and slowly became more and more orange over the years – the equivalent of going grey in the car-ageing process. It was a source of much mirth at vet school because I stubbornly refused to acknowledge that it was orange. To me it was red, because that was its colour when it arrived. I loved that car. My mother had won it in a competition at the Castleford branch of Asda many years earlier. It was an incredibly complicated competition but the winner from each Asda store in the country received a brand-new Mini Metro. My sister, Kate, and I shared the car when we were sixth-formers, and then I inherited it for my trips to and from university, and to get me to the various vet practices that I had to visit. It never failed me, although I did periodically have to reach out of the window to make the windscreen wipers work.

My interview at Skeldale was not like most job interviews. There were no chairs, no questions like 'Where do you see yourself in five or ten years' time?' or 'What are your thoughts on the government's policies on tuberculosis control?' Instead I had a prolonged and rambling chat with the partners, Jim, Peter and Tim. Jim is the son of Alf Wight, and he wanted to reduce his hours at the practice to enable him to write a book about his father's life. Our interviews for new vets are still like this – disorganized and rambling – but we usually find the right person for the job, and it worked on this occasion. We quickly realized that we were mutually suited.

And so it started, my veterinary career at the most famous veterinary practice in the world – though first, I had a stint in Caithness to get through …

2

Anthrax and Appendicitis in Scotland

The day after graduation I was back in my reddish-orange Mini Metro, rushing up the A1 (the car could do that bit by itself), across the Pennines this time, to be the best man at the wedding that followed the aforementioned stag party in the Peak District. One of my best mates from university, Pete, was marrying Rachel, the girl he had met in our very first term at Pembroke, six years before. It was a great day and the first of many weddings that would punctuate my weekends, when not on call, over the first few years of life as a newly qualified vet. But there was no time for rest. I had less than twenty-four hours to get to the most remote and northerly part of the United Kingdom to my first job, as a locum veterinary surgeon, in Thurso, Caithness. I would be here for eight weeks before starting at the Skeldale practice in Thirsk.

I had been to the Scottish surgery several times as a student. I would spend three or four weeks at a time there, seeing practice, and

I loved the people, the area and the way of life. The first time I visited this place, it was with my girlfriend, Anne. We saw practice there together for six fabulous weeks during the summer before Anne's final year and my penultimate year at vet school. We stayed in a tiny tent in a cliff top campsite about half a mile from the practice, so it was really part work and part holiday. The staff at the practice thought it was a strange coincidence that two students from the same vet school should both arrive in this desolate part of the country at the same time. Not many students would venture to such a far-flung corner of the country, and initially they had no idea that we were an item. This misunderstanding was quickly rectified when, one evening after a meal in the local restaurant (there was only one restaurant in Thurso and it fitted all purposes – Italian on Monday, Indian on Tuesday, Chinese on Wednesday and Thursday and then 'normal' for the rest of the week), we were spotted entwined in a romantic embrace by the phone box. Eyebrows were raised over coffee the next morning and the record was set straight. There was also some astonishment that we were camping in Caithness, as there were generally horizontal winds, more often than not accompanied by horizontal rain. We were, however, blessed with the best summer there had been for many years. While it wasn't exactly shorts weather, our tent on the cliff top remained dry, and didn't disappear out to sea in a gale.

It was a wonderful place to learn the ropes. The vets there worked harder than any I have ever met. To calve five cows in an evening would not be unusual. I particularly admired a gruff veterinary surgeon called Frank. He was usually averse to taking students with him, maybe because of the danger of them dying of Benson & Hedges intoxication in his car, but he and I got on well. I asked him one evening, as we headed out on a visit to see a cow with a prolapsed uterus, how long the buzz associated with being on call would last? He pulled heavily on his Benson & Hedges before narrowing his eyes (as he always did before saying something – maybe to keep the smoke out), 'Aye, it took me about twenty ...' and then he paused. I waited for the next word to be 'weeks' or 'months' but, as he puffed out smoke, 'years' was the next thing he said. I remember, at that point, thinking that this career was definitely going to be more of a way of life than a job.

Frank was an inspirational teacher and I admired him immensely. As a student he gave me my first opportunity to perform a caesarean section on a cow, and I remember every incision and every suture of that first epic piece of surgery. The cow was old, black and very thin, and she was heavily in calf. She was clearly at the point of calving but could not muster the energy to do it by herself. The prognosis was poor and she evidently needed a caesarean to have any chance of saving both her and her calf. The problem was that it seemed unreasonable to charge the farmer the full cost of the operation when the outlook was so gloomy.

As Frank drew heavily on his B&H, he pondered the options for the cow. He made a suggestion that made the hairs on the back of my neck rise. 'I'll tell you what,' he proposed to the farmer, 'we'll let the student do it, and we won't charge you for the operation.'

Frank instructed me from the comfort of a rusty gate while continuing to puff on his cigarette. I completed the surgery without complication and as I walked off the farm, I felt ten feet tall. Frank had given me this amazing first opportunity and I was, and still am, so grateful. I'm still not sure, though, if it was simply to give him a chance to finish his cigarette uninterrupted!

While I was at the practice as a student, I sometimes stayed with another of the vets, called Willy. Willy was a quiet and calm man who spoke slowly and gently and loved hill walking, and very old Scottish single malt whisky. He, too, was very hard working, and would punctuate his busy days by calling at a nearby beach to walk his spaniel, Gyp. The beaches around Thurso are spectacular and even a fifteen-minute walk would clear the mind like nothing else. In fact it was to this particular beach that I would return, six months later, as a newly qualified veterinary surgeon, to contemplate whether my embryonic career was about to come to a premature end.

It was the second week of my locum job in Thurso and I had thrown myself into the job with enthusiasm. Cattle and sheep were everywhere and it was the perfect place to start a veterinary career. I would get ample experience very quickly. I also reasoned that when I left after this short-term post, I could leave any early mistakes 600 miles behind me, when I got to Thirsk two months later. I had put my initials next to two visits in the day book on the morning in question (this was, and still is, the way to sign up to a job). The first call was to a cow with mastitis. The second was to a stirk (a young bovine somewhere between a calf and an adult), which had died suddenly. We had been taught at vet school that, in cases of sudden death, a tiny blood sample needed to be taken from the ear, avoiding any spillage or exposure to the air. The blood sample then had to be examined under a microscope, before a post mortem could be performed. This was to check for the presence of anthrax bacilli in the carcass. To do a full post mortem would inevitably cause anthrax to be exposed to the air, which would result in spores contaminating the environment, triggering a major disease outbreak. Although the practice had not seen any recent outbreaks of the disease, it was reasonably close to a place called Gruinyard Island, the site of secret testing of the deadly anthrax bacteria when it was being considered as an agent for 'germ warfare' in the Second World War. Anthrax was certainly something I needed to check for and this needed to be done on the farm before I could get on with a full post mortem.

As I packed the practice microscope and was about to head out of the door, a colleague, also very experienced and keen on dermatology, called me back. He needed the microscope to analyse a complicated skin case later that morning. He assured me that there would be no need to test for anthrax but, if I deemed it necessary when I had seen the dead beast, I should take a sample of blood and analyse it later at the practice. I bowed to his seniority and experience and was reassured by his advice not to worry about such a rare condition. I clambered into the practice van and was soon on my way.

I arrived at the farm to see the dead animal lying limp, next to a midden heap. It had a small amount of frothy blood at its nostrils. I chatted with the farmer who told me that it had been perfectly normal the previous evening. Keen to establish the cause of death, I set about a post mortem examination, closely inspecting all the body systems and taking numerous samples for analysis, which I put in a big plastic bag. 'Blimey, that's a large spleen,' I remember thinking, as I explored the blood-filled abdomen. Before I left, I had a look at the other animals in the same group. Most of them had very high temperatures, but few other signs of illness. I was sure my thorough post mortem would give me the answers.

As I drove back to the practice, my mind was racing with all the possible diagnoses and I started to wonder if I should, after all, have done that anthrax test.

I went past the beach where Willy and I had walked his dog earlier that year, and pulled into the carpark nearby so I could collect my thoughts and check my textbook. I looked up the signs of anthrax: no rigor mortis, blood at the mouth, copious internal bleeding, large spleen, very high temperatures in other animals, and sudden death. I started to feel sick as I stared at the bag of bits, on the passenger seat next to me in my little van. As I flicked through the pages of the book, my face started to itch all over. I peered into the rearview mirror of the van to see angry, red wheals all over my forehead and cheeks. The final point on the list of signs of anthrax, which I read in horror, stated: 'skin lesions in humans who have been exposed, followed by rapid and sudden death'. By now I was certain that not only my veterinary career but also my life was about to be cut short. I went for a brief walk along this lovely beach, thinking that, since it was probably my last, I may as well enjoy it.

Forty-five minutes later I was at the local veterinary laboratory. They cheerfully confirmed that the animal had died from acute pneumonia and there was not a trace of anthrax in the specimens. But what of my skin lesions – surely they were evidence that I had contracted the deadly disease? No – I had spent an hour stooped over the dead animal right next to a muck heap, swarming with infamous Scottish midges. They had enjoyed a feast on my juicy English skin!

So I lived to fight another day, a little the wiser.

The rest of my time at Thurso was less eventful. I developed a sound grounding for my new career and a healthy respect for the animals with which I would be dealing. On one occasion I went to see a cow, which the farmer described as simply being 'off colour'. These cases are both easy and difficult. Easy because the farmer doesn't know what is wrong with his animal, so I might have a better than average chance of impressing him with my diagnosis, but difficult because I would have no real clues to go on. Cows in this part of the world were not always amenable to a thorough examination. Luckily for me, I had enthusiasm and naïvity on my side. So, as the two farmers tried to catch the cow, which had not been handled for six months, I felt sure I would be able to ascertain its problems. Thirty minutes later, the cow had been lassoed. After a basic examination, during which I failed to elucidate the cause of its problems, I explained in detail to the two weather-worn Scots that I was intending to place a needle into the animal's abdomen to take a sample of abdominal fluid. The farmers looked at each other with wry smiles, fully aware of what was going to happen next. I was blissfully unaware of what was going to happen. I can only imagine what did happen, because whatever it was, it left me ten feet away, lying on my back in the straw with stars spinning in front of my eyes, a bloodied nose and a very sore head. I had not succeeded in sampling the cow's abdominal fluid and I decided that, on balance, it was probably not necessary, or indeed possible. I avoided a trip to hospital on that occasion, but not so the following week.

When the afternoon's work had been completed, the staff at the practice all retired home for tea at about 5 p.m., before returning for evening surgery at half past six. We would often have tea at each other's houses to chat about the day. Willy, a bachelor, and I would often have tea together but one day it was not as relaxing as it could have been. Poor Willy had been ill all day and had developed a severe bout of abdominal pain. In hindsight this was not altogether surprising because Willy's diet consisted almost entirely of potatoes and meat pies. During my time in Thurso, sharing Willy's house, I never once saw a vegetable nor a piece of salad pass his lips. He looked more and more pale and weak as the day wore on, so we decided he should go to the local hospital to see a doctor. It must have been pretty serious, because vets usually treat any minor ailments themselves.

I bundled him into the van and drove him the thirty minutes to the outpatients department at Wick Hospital. After a brief assessment, Willy was admitted to the ward. I was presumed to be a close relative, and was ushered to his bedside. A nurse came to put him on a drip. As vets, we do this all the time, and it is sometimes hard to stop our patients from chewing the catheter, but Willy was not in any position to object to his drip in any way. He looked very sick.

After about half an hour, a diminutive doctor appeared and carefully explained to Willy that he needed to perform an 'internal examination'. As the doctor donned his rubber gloves, the look on Willy's face changed from one of weak pallor to one of panic and fear, and I thought he was going to rip his drip line out and run out of the ward. Willy would have performed this procedure thousands of times on his patients, both canine and bovine, but suddenly it didn't seem at all appropriate. He was on the receiving end! I could not stop fits of hysterical laughter welling up and, with tears streaming from my eyes, I rushed out to sit in the corridor. I must have looked distraught, as I sat convulsing in the corridor with tears in my eyes, holding my head in my hands. A helpful nurse was walking past. She had seen us when we arrived and she reassuringly patted me on the back. 'Don't worry,' she soothed. 'Your boyfriend is going to be fine.'

Soon afterwards, I left this desolate but beautiful area, armed with stories, experience and confidence and excited to be starting my new job in the equally beautiful North York Moors, in the market town of Thirsk.

3

'Job's a Bad Un'

After finishing in Thurso and before starting in Thirsk, my little reddish-orange Metro had one last mission. During my final year at vet school, I had received a bursary from the British Cattle Veterinary Association to undertake a research project, supported by the ever-calm and inspirational Dr Jackson. One of his areas of expertise was bovine obstetrics. We had devised a project to measure the oxygenation levels of calves during labour. This is done routinely in babies but veterinary medicine was lagging some way behind. During the project, I had been the first person to use this technique in calves and lambs and had written a paper setting out my findings. It was published in the *Veterinary Record*, our professional journal, while I was still a student. I had been invited to present my paper to a meeting of the BCVA in Exeter, Devon. I was in Thurso, Caithness. My little car had to make it pretty much from John O'Groats to Land's End. I had to give my talk and then get back up to Yorkshire for the first day of my new job. My car and I made it, but only just.

Starting at Skeldale Veterinary Centre could not have been more straightforward. I already had some basic skills, which I had learnt in Scotland, and I was sharing a house with my university friend, Jon (he of the moustache). He had been at Skeldale as a student and, since two posts had arisen at about the same time, the partners had decided to employ both of us. Jon had started soon after graduation while I had been in Scotland, so he was familiar with some of the peculiarities of the area and the practice.

My first night on call was particularly memorable. It was also my very first night at the practice – there was no time for easing in gradually. After evening surgery had finished, I was sent out to see a ewe with orf. Orf is a viral infection that affects sheep, giving them painful, crusty swellings on the mouth and face. It can also affect the udder, so little lambs can catch it from their mothers and the sores make it painful for them when they try to suck. It is straightforward to diagnose and the treatment, while mainly symptomatic rather than curative, is simple. It was an easy first job for my first night on call. At about eight o'clock, the beeper went off again. In those days, mobile phones were not widely used so, when this happened, we had to find a telephone box, or borrow the phone of whichever farm we happened to be at or near. There was a cow to see with mastitis. The farmer had noticed it during evening milking. I took directions and went straight there. The farmer was a chap called Colin. He lived in the small village of Thirlby, which nestled in a very sheltered spot just below Sutton Bank. From his yard, you can see the white stone cliff from which the bigger village of Sutton-under-Whitestonecliffe gets its name. On this autumn evening, the bright limestone reflected the orange sunset and it looked spectacular. Colin came out to show me the cow. She had nasty mastitis. Her udder was massively swollen and she had a very high temperature. Mastitis in cows can usually be treated with antibiotic injections and intra-mammary tubes (tubes of antibiotics which are instilled into the udder via the teat). However, in this case the infection was too severe for this simple remedy, in part because the teat was blocked. The skin of the udder was tight and purple and without aggressive treatment there was a high risk of necrosis and then gangrene. This is very serious and leaves an enormous messy and smelly problem for weeks. I decided that the proper course of action was to take my scalpel and lance the udder, as if it were a huge abscess. As I explained my plan to Colin, I could see he wasn't convinced. 'Can yer not give her an injection then, Vetnery?' he asked.

I noticed that some of his family had arrived in the gloomy cow byre. It was as if the whole family had come to coerce me into a more benign course of treatment. The last to arrive was Colin's striking daughter, who was about eighteen. She had a shock of red hair and a very short nightie, made somewhat incongruous by knee-high wellies. I was somewhat flummoxed at the arrival of this siren, who had surely come along to distract me from the task in hand. I regathered my thoughts and made preparations for my bold incision. Sure enough, a river of fetid pus came spewing out of the cow's udder, all over the floor and all over my Wellington boots. I felt quite pleased that my actions had been justified, as there were gasps of awe from the onlookers. I finally returned home, well after dark, and recounted the tale of my first evening on call to my housemate and colleague Jon, including the arrival of the red-headed siren.

'D'you know what?' he said, as he opened a bottle of beer, 'the very same thing happened to me on my first night on call!' We both chuckled.

*

At that time it was easy to gain, or lose, a reputation. It was a small community and gossip spread quickly. The arrival of two new young vets was unusual, especially since we were both the same age and of a similar disposition. Clients would often mistake us for the other one and we would sometimes play on this, especially if a case was not going to plan.

We were soon signed up to Ampleforth village cricket team, and played in the Ryedale evening league. Games would take us to villages further afield than our usual patch. We played one game on a beautiful ground in the garden of an enormous house called Hovingham Hall, on its front lawn. It was reputed to be the favourite cricket ground of the famous Fred Trueman. We felt honoured, because there could be no better person to judge it as the best. Not all pitches were of that quality, though. At the other end of the spectrum, the infamous 'Spout House' was almost impossible to play cricket on. Not only was it on an incredible slope, but the outfield was littered with both cow pats and actual sheep. Fielders had to be arranged along one boundary alone, at the bottom of the hill.

Games were usually played in spring and summer in the evenings and consisted of sixteen eight-ball overs for each team. It was always a rush to get to the venue after evening surgery and it was a standing joke: 'Vet's late again.' Since it was unusual that we could both play in the same game, as one of us was invariably on duty, the team sheet would simply say 'Vet' and either Jon or I would take the place. The captain, Mike Dobson, would not usually know which of us was going to appear.

Neither of us was particularly talented at cricket but what we lacked in ability, we made up for in enthusiasm. We were certainly the most active and mobile in the outfield. Mind you, being active in the field was important, mainly to keep warm. In one early season game, the outfield was covered in snow.

Jon was a 'Michael Vaughan' kind of batsman, upright and technically precise. When he did make contact, he had a glorious cover drive. I, on the other hand, was more like a talentless version of Ian Botham. I would both bowl and bat, neither particularly well, although the high point of my short cricketing career was a 50 not out, and then two wickets in my first over. We had our own Fred Trueman, too, in the form of a massive farmer called Clive. He always opened the bowling, and when he was bowling we had a deep fine leg and a very fine third man to back up the creaking wicket keeper. Clive's cricket season always ended early when he had to concentrate on getting the harvest in, from mid summer. Whatever the result, we would convene in the nearest pub for sandwiches and beer. The post match chat was always more important than the score.

We ate a lot of sandwiches in those days. It was a hungry business being a young vet. At lunchtimes, we had a habit of buying a large loaf of 'Country Crunch' from the bakers, as we lived close to the surgery and could easily go home for lunch. Without any discussion as to which of us would buy the loaf, our system seemed to work. The worst outcome was that we would end up with two loaves but since we ate voraciously, this did not present a problem. One day, the shop was particularly busy. I took my place at the back of the queue and had not been waiting long before one of the shop staff shouted, at the top of her voice, across the packed shop, 'It's OK, your friend has already been in to collect it already!'

A few months in and I thought my reputation as a decent vet

was developing well. However, one evening it took something of a battering.

It was a Saturday night in mid winter, cold and very dark, when I was called to a local dairy farm. A cow was having difficulty calving. I had not been to this farm before and so I took detailed notes on how to get there and sped off at high speed. Calvings are always an emergency and tensions often run high, with farmers anxious about the outcome for both the cow and the calf. I arrived in the pitch-black yard, and eventually found the farmer, Steve, in the cow shed, already with his arm where mine should have been. 'Ah've just about got this un,' he grunted. It looked hard work, but Steve managed to deliver the calf, which, sadly, showed no signs of life. It was disappointing, but the calf had clearly been dead for some time and the outcome was nobody's fault.

We looked at each other. I seemed somewhat redundant, but I offered to check the cow out for injuries or other problems, and to check for a second calf. It was what we had been taught to do. *Always* check for a second calf, or a third lamb. I felt smug as I quickly identified the presence of a twin. It became apparent that it was breach, that is, coming tail first, with both back legs pointing forwards towards the cow's head. It is impossible for the calf to be born by itself in this presentation. The back legs need to be manipulated so they are pointing backwards, which then allows it to be delivered. All went according to plan. I repositioned the calf and pulled it out, much to everyone's delight. The newborn, however, was not at all well. Its breathing was shallow and erratic and it looked close to death. I had a plan. I knew all about neonatal acidosis – my recent research project had been related to this topic, so I felt it was my area of expertise. I rushed to my car boot to get a vial of some powder which I knew would counteract the acidosis that I presumed was the cause of this calf's problems. I explained my plan and administered the treatment. In my mind, the calf was going to splutter, lift its head and rise like Lazarus. I stood back, awaiting the miracle. Sadly, a miracle did not occur. The calf did indeed splutter, but then promptly expired. Suddenly the cow shed became silent. It was pretty silent before, actually, but I expected to see one of those tumbleweeds rolling through, as the atmosphere became leaden. We stood staring at a healthy cow, but two dead calves.

'Well. Job's a bad un!' Steve blurted out, and stumped off back to his house, leaving me cold and traumatized in his cow shed. I had no torch and the lights had been turned off, so it took me several miserable minutes, avoiding farmyard obstacles and sleeping cows, before I could find my way back to the car and make a hasty retreat. My first visit to one of the practice's biggest farm clients had been an unmitigated disaster. I got home and gloomily went straight to bed, feeling very dejected.

I slept soundly, despite the spectre of my beeper, which usually led to a broken night's sleep, even if no calls came through. Early the following morning, I got a message to say there was an urgent call to see a foal with a laceration on its nose. The owner was very upset and so I rushed off, again, eager to get there as soon as I could. The visit was in the opposite direction to the previous night's call, but I found my way there without any problem. A young lady, about my age, was there, holding the young foal. I opened the gate to the yard, hoping to make a good impression.

'Oh no, not you!' she said, which surprised me because I couldn't recall meeting her before and certainly could not think of a reason why she should react quite so vehemently. I examined the injury and explained that it needed stitches.

'Well, let's hope you do a better job than you did on that calf last night,' she grumbled.

'Oh my God!' I thought. Less than twelve hours had elapsed and now the whole of Yorkshire knew how rubbish I was. How could that have happened? The girl did not let on how she knew and I chose not to pursue this line of discussion. Rather, I concentrated on my local anaesthetic and making tidy sutures.

It was only two weeks later when I went back to remove the sutures, the wound having healed beautifully, that I plucked up courage to find out how she knew about the demise of the calf.

'I'm Steve's girlfriend,' she explained.

'Phew,' I thought.

4

There's Nowt Better than a Good Old Cow!

During our first few months at Thirsk, there was one local farmer who became hugely important to Jon and me. She and her husband had a small and very traditional dairy herd, just on the outskirts of town and about quarter of a mile from our house. Jeanie and Steve had devoted their lives to rearing their stock and milking their cows twice a day and had been doing this for the last fifty years. The cows came wandering in each milking time, taking their own places in the byre, where they were fastened side by side. They were creatures of habit as much as their owners.

We would often be called early in the morning. Steve and Jeanie rose at 4.30 each morning and expected us to do the same if one of their animals was sick – usually a cow that was struggling to calve or a case of milk fever. Milk fever is a condition whereby the blood level of calcium drops, soon after calving time. This leads to muscular weakness and the cow becomes initially wobbly and then, quite quickly, recumbent. Although it is easily identified and treated, it can develop into a serious condition in just a few hours, so it is always treated as an emergency. Since it was usually noticed early in the morning, at the time of milking, we would usually be called around 5 a.m. to attend to such cases. At this time the practice served about fifty family-run dairy herds. Sometimes the poor cows were in a terrible mess, having slipped during the night due to the muscle weakness that developed as the blood calcium dropped. They might have been stuck in mud or slurry for a while, so rectifying the problem was often a messy and dirty affair. Luckily, when such a call came from Steve and Jeanie, the cows were never messy or dirty as they had huge, thick straw beds, and were always scrupulously clean. In many ways the cattle were treated as members of the family and Jeanie could often be heard shouting down the cow byre as she turned them out to grass, 'There's nowt better than a good old cow!'

Since the farm was so close to our house, we could be home within half an hour with a bacon sandwich and a cup of tea to recharge before the actual day of work began.

Jeanie was a somewhat eccentric lady, with hair and eyes pointing in all directions. She was well known around the market square and in the auction mart as she was born and bred in Thirsk, like many in this rural community. She was very kind and would always give a home to stray or feral kittens that arrived, injured or otherwise, at the practice, cheerfully calling 'Happy to help out, son!' as she shuffled out of the practice. The cats that she adopted had a great life on her farm. They were treated like royalty, and the farmhouse kitchen must have sometimes had a dozen cats in various states of relaxation about the room. In return for these cats, Jeanie would bring in large containers of sweets of all descriptions. Sometimes Liquorice Allsorts or boiled sweets in large plastic jars, or sometimes a selection of the wrapped variety. Either way, they were copious and ubiquitous. There were many myths about the source of these sweets, but their provenance, to this day, remains obscure.

As two young male vets, Jeanie took something of a maternal shine to us. She went out of her way to ensure we had sustenance greater than just boiled sweets. During evening surgery, messages would appear in the day book, not of pneumonic calves in urgent need of attention, or ewes struggling to lamb, but messages that read: 'Send 'em round. I've got 'em a pie.'

Sure enough, whichever of us was first to leave would call at Stoneybrough Farm on our way home and pick up our tea. Jeanie was an expert pie maker. Her speciality was meat and potato. Meat and juices would spill out of the sides of these great constructions, always sitting in a white and blue enamel pie dish. We got into a perfect routine of returning one empty pie dish, only to replace it with another, bursting with ingredients.

Occasionally we would be lucky and receive a curd tart – a Yorkshire speciality made of milk, raisins and nutmeg. Jeanie's were remarkable because they were made with 'beastlings'. The message in the day book might read: 'Julian, call at Jeanie's. She's made you a beastlings pie.' As a young vet, I was unfamiliar with some of the local dialect, and I was not acquainted with the word 'beastlings'. I have to say it did not sound an appetizing treat. I had visions of small, dead animals and eyeballs peering out of the pastry. Later that evening, without the help of internet searches, I ascertained that 'beastlings' was the local term used to describe colostrum. This is the first milk that a cow produces after she has calved. It is thick and creamy and full of protein. It gives the calf a good start in life, as it coats its intestines with protective antibodies. After a good helping of Jeanie's pie, I felt safe in the knowledge that my bowels were bursting with antibodies and that I could withstand any gastro-intestinal challenge.

In those days, being a young vet, visiting the many local family farms could be as much a gastronomic journey as it was a professional one. There were two other farms where there would always be a feast. The first was Scawlings Farm in Oldstead, a small, pretty village just round the corner from the famous White Horse of Kilburn. The White Horse was carved out of the cliff above the village of the same name, by a local school teacher with his pupils, in 1857. It can be seen from all over this part of Yorkshire and, reputedly, from as far away as Lincolnshire. On the days when I visited Scawlings Farm, I passed right under the feet of the horse, although the view of it from close up was less spectacular.

This dairy farm was the first I visited when I started in Thirsk. On my very first morning, Peter Wright, the senior partner, asked me how I was at PDs. 'PD' is short for pregnancy diagnosis and in this case he was referring to pregnancy diagnosis in cattle. This involves palpating the cow's uterus, via the rectum. The procedure is not at all painful for the cow and allows an examination of as much of the cow's abdomen as we can reach. A rectal examination is a crucial part of a large animal vet's job, as this way we can palpate the ovaries, left kidney, uterus, the cervix, bladder, rumen and other bits. It is an important thing to be able to do with confidence, but it can take some time before a newly graduated veterinary surgeon becomes fully accomplished in this task. In the case of a PD, we were specifically feeling the uterus to ascertain if the cow was pregnant. We could also give some information about the stage of pregnancy. An early pregnancy would feel like a small water-filled balloon in the uterine horn. A later pregnancy would feel like a football and later still we would palpate a whole foetus, and by its size, be able to give an idea of its age. Brimming with confidence, I assured Pete I would have absolutely no trouble with a morning of PDs. Astonishingly, he was happy to accept my assertion, and allowed me to launch myself into the task, without supervision from a more experienced vet.

We made regular, often twice-weekly visits to Scawlings Farm so I quickly became accustomed to the bumpy road to Oldstead, and good friends with the farmer, Howard. He had a dairy herd of about eighty cows, all high yielders with great genetic merit. Howard had signed up to a scheme, set up by the practice, whereby dairy farmers would pay the practice a set monthly fee based on the number of cows they owned and, in return, would receive as many visits as necessary. It was a scheme years ahead of its time, but had been badly miscalculated by Mr Sinclair, its instigator (Siegfried Farnon in the Herriot books), so the practice lost money hand over fist. Luckily only two dairy farms were signed up to this scheme, and wily Howard was one of them. I wouldn't say he took unfair advantage of the deal but he certainly got more than his money's worth. He clearly saw the benefits of a young and enthusiastic vet and 'free' visits and I spent a lot of time on his farm. I still remember visiting his farm five times on one Sunday in winter to treat a downer cow. Consequently we became great friends and I honed my large animal skills on his cows.

I would usually arrive to do the routine fertility visits at about 9.30 in the morning and, after inspecting about ten cows, Howard's wife, Chris, would appear with steaming mugs of coffee, flapjacks, parkin and biscuits. We would stop what we were doing and, often without even bothering to wash our hands, tuck into the spread. It was very welcome as it was invariably cold at Scawlings Farm.

The other farm that had a great reputation for providing an amazing spread of food was nearby to Howard's. The farm had a beef suckler herd. This type of herd differs from a dairy herd, in that the cows are not milked. The calves suckle the cows directly and grow into beasts that will ultimately end up as a Sunday roast. The cows usually calve in either spring or autumn (spring was more popular in and around Thirsk) and then spend all summer out in the fields, the cows eating grass, and the calves suckling milk and also eating grass when they get bigger. Suckler herds were very different from dairy herds from a practice perspective because, rather than visiting them twice a week, we would often visit them only a few times each year, for difficult calvings, or to see calves that were poorly with scour (diarrhoea), pneumonia or other ailments. A visit from a vet was regarded as a special occasion.

In those days, cattle needed to be tested for two diseases, tuberculosis and brucellosis, under the auspices of MAFF (the Ministry of Agriculture, Fisheries and Food) who oversaw disease control in the country. Tuberculosis testing was, in those days, every three years and brucellosis testing (which was a blood test) happened every two years. This meant that even farms that had very few problems and little requirement for a vet would still have us visit on an approximately annual basis.

This particular farm had about forty cows and, as far as I can remember, we only ever visited them to do a statutory TB or brucellosis test. Consequently the handling facilities were somewhat antediluvian. What should have been a straightforward visit of a couple of hours would inevitably turn into one that took all day. On my first visit to the farm, I had to do both tests together. When it fell to do both tests on the same day, the time it took was approximately doubled, since we had to take a blood sample from a vein in the cow's tail, and then move round to the neck to do the intradermal skin test for TB. In the TB test, tiny amounts of avian and bovine tuberculin are injected into the skin on the neck. In essence, if a lumpy swelling develops at the site of the bovine tuberculin injection, but not at the site of the avian tuberculin, then the cow is likely to have TB. This test was invented shortly after the Second World War and is still generally regarded as the most reliable test for identifying TB reactors. However, since the ministry's policy of test and cull that has been in place for all this time has not changed the incidence of TB in cattle, it does raise questions over the efficacy of the scheme.

I donned my wellies and, as always, gave them a scrub to make sure they were clean and that I was not transferring any diseases from farm to farm (I was in the habit of scrubbing my boots before I left each farm and also as soon as I arrived on another). I met the farmer and we wandered around the corner of the shed to see the handling arrangement. This was the moment I would get the first clue as to how long the morning's work would take. A good system could save a couple of hours. A bad system might mean the job would take all day. In this case, my heart sank as I saw the creaking cattle crush, tilted against a wall for support. To make matters worse it was surrounded by thick mud. It was the type of mud that was very hard to move around in and made it almost impossible to make a quick getaway from a fast-moving cow. Thick mud that worked its way up the inside of your waterproof trousers all the way to your crotch. It was slow and laborious work and it did indeed, as predicted, take most of the day.

Sweaty and muddy, I finished the job and headed into the farmhouse to complete my paperwork. Work for the ministry always required copious amounts of form-filling. I could not believe my eyes when I saw the farmhouse kitchen, with its stone-flagged floor and roaring fire. The enormous table was covered in food of all types and descriptions, like a medieval banquet. Tongue sandwiches, fruitcake, biscuits, apple pies, cheese, tea in a pot with a knitted tea cosy. I had never met these folks before, but they invited me into their home as if I were a long-lost cousin. As I made my way back to the practice after lunch (or what was now half way between lunch and tea), I had forgotten all about the tenacity of the mud, or the stubborn refusal of the cows to enter the crush, and I felt sure I would be signing up to do their next test.

Not all farms were as accommodating to our needs. I can recall one particular day (actually two days, because it took so long) when I was castrating young bulls. This was the job that nobody rushed to do. It was very physical and required either removing the testicles using a sharp scalpel blade, or 'nipping' them, by using a set of clamps called Burdizzos. These are applied to the spermatic cord and crush the blood vessels supplying the testicles. Without their blood supply, the testicles quickly shrivel, so male cattle do not act as bulls. The castrated animals are much safer to handle than bulls, and are more amenable to being farmed. While the procedure is not particularly painful to the cattle, it nearly always results in kicks and bruises to the veterinary surgeon, for whom the procedure is, therefore, often very painful. Consequently, there was never a queue of vets waiting to sign up to this job. On this occasion, I had about eighty to do. They were around ten months old and each one weighed at least 400 kilograms. Oh, and they weren't used to being handled because they had spent the whole of their life, so far, in a field.

My job for the day was to capture these wild animals, usher them into a pen then persuade them into a long race – a sort of fenced corridor – along the side of an enormous cattle shed, where I could castrate them. It was raining, and the guttering along the edge of the shed was broken, so there was a steady stream of water pouring onto the bulls and onto me. At the same time as I was castrating these bulls, the farmer, a strong rugby-playing chap called Steve, was putting slow-release mineral boluses down their throats. This was to provide minerals over a long period to ensure that they stayed healthy. It was a good opportunity to get both jobs done at once, as these cattle did not go into the race or the crush very often.

We were slowly making our way through the large pen of robust cattle. At about midday, the farmer put down his bolusing gun and hopped onto his quad bike.

'Right then, I'll be off,' he announced.

All I could think to say was, 'Oh!' and then, 'What, now?' as I peered into the pen.

We still had plenty to do.

'I'll be back after me dinner,' he said and, before I could protest, he whizzed off and left me under a spout of rain.

I plodded on for about an hour, working singlehandedly, castrating and administering the boluses, until he returned to help with the rest of the job.

Eventually, we got to the end. This time, not with muddy trousers, but with soaking wet trousers and soaking wet everything else. There was no full table of food in a toasty farmhouse kitchen.

I resolved, 'Next time, this is Jon's job.'

5

The Evil Salve

The 1990s was a difficult time for the veterinary profession and the cattle industry. Not because I had been let loose on the veterinary world, but because it was struggling with the legacy of BSE (bovine spongiform encephalopathy), a terrible and frightening disease that had a devastating effect on everyone involved. Its colloquial name, 'mad cow disease', was perfectly apt.

It was terrible and frightening because it was a new disease. Nothing like it had been seen before in cattle, and nobody could understand how it was spread or from where it came. Its effects on affected animals were dramatic and often dangerous. It had a rapid course and would strike down adult cattle, predominantly dairy cows, in their prime. The signs would progress quickly to severe neurological disease and cows would literally 'go mad' – become uncoordinated, kick out and behave with uncharacteristic aggression.

It took everyone by surprise. An experienced veterinary surgeon called David Bee, working in Petersfield, Hampshire was one of the first people to suggest that the country might be dealing with a new disease. He was one of those endlessly enthusiastic vets with boundless energy and a career's worth of knowledge. My wife, Anne, spent much of the formative part of her training under his expert tutorship.

BSE had many similarities to a neurological disease called Scrapie, seen in sheep, and this was eventually identified as the original source of the new disease. The rules governing the way animal by-products were handled had been changed and the result was that contaminated sheep meat ended up in cattle food (a disturbing thought, even without its implications for disease). Since this was mainly used in the dairy sector, rather than in beef herds, it was dairy cows that bore the brunt of the epidemic.

Even more alarming was the appearance, admittedly at a low level, of a human version of the same condition, called 'new variant CJD' (new variant Creutzfeldt-Jakob disease). This was a fatal and dramatic brain disease and there was no way of knowing how many people would contract it and if it was, indeed, transmitted from contaminated beef products. Quite rightly, massive restrictions were imposed on the sale of British beef. Looking back, it is astonishing that the cattle industry managed to survive such a monumental crisis. Calves were immediately worthless and it became routine to have dairy bull calves shot at birth, as they could not be used in any way. Beef exports were banned, as was beef on the bone, and all cattle over thirty months of age were banned from entering the food chain. These animals would be killed and incinerated. Everyone was paranoid about any cow that even so much as twitched her ears in an odd way. It was a depressing time for everyone.

I remember, one afternoon, being called to see a heifer that was doing just that – twitching her ears in a peculiar way. It was not a classic clinical sign of BSE, but we were very tuned to subtle changes in the behaviour of cows that might intimate the disease. I was immediately suspicious and called the ministry, which was standard procedure in these cases. If the ministry vet then considered the animal likely to be infected with BSE, it would be euthanased by injection and the brain would be analysed. The ministry vet came and looked at the heifer, and quickly confirmed the condition, leaving me with a large bottle of blue pentobarbitone – a very strong barbiturate that we used for euthanasia. The farmer was clearly distraught at the loss of one of his best young animals, but worse, she was in calf and due to calve any day. We discussed the options and I decided to perform a 'bush caesarean'. This is a caesarean section whereby the sole purpose is to save the life of the calf at the expense of the mother, usually because the mother is terminally ill. In this case, I would take the calf out and then inject the BSE-affected dam. I sought confirmation from the ministry vet, who was reluctant to authorize it, but clearly would turn a blind eye for the sake of saving the calf.

'Just be careful,' were his parting words. 'We don't know anything about this bloody disease and you are about to delve your arms right into her abdomen and uterus. Make sure you wear some gloves!' It had never occurred to me that there might be a reasonable risk of contracting the disease myself from the heifer. There was a much more obvious danger: infected animals would charge, kick and behave in a generally aggressive and unpredictable manner, so there was a real risk of being badly injured. It did, however, go as well as could be expected under the miserable circumstances. I removed a healthy female calf without injury or accident and, as far as I could tell, avoided ingesting any blood or other fluids. I glumly euthanased her mother and left, in the darkness, very dejected.

By this time, some idea about the pathogenesis of the disease was developing. It was found to be transmitted not by a conventional infectious agent like a bacterium or a virus, but something much smaller and altogether more simple – a protein. The individual agent was called a 'prion', an infectious protein, and while it was not fully understood, the general consensus among the scientific community was that, in simple terms, cattle had been fed the brains of scrapie-infected sheep, exposing them to this infectious protein. This then crossed from one species to another to cause a new disease. In the farming community, however, without the benefit of laboratory tests and scientific papers, everyone had their own theories. A popular one revolved around the use of organophosphate insecticide treatments, used to prevent insect bites and other parasitic diseases. While these were very effective and used quite extensively, most farmers really disliked them and sensed that they were not very safe. Now, happily, these insecticides are banned; even if they weren't responsible for BSE, they were fairly toxic compounds. It was a standing but not very funny joke among farmers that the people employed as crop sprayers did not enjoy a long life.

One of the oldest clients of the practice, a Mr Norris, had his own theory about the origins of BSE. It is documented in a series of five short letters, which he addressed to 'The Vets' and delivered, by hand, to the surgery in the late 1980s. These letters still reside in a small and faded brown envelope on the bottom shelf of the cabinet, in an upstairs room in our current surgery at Skeldale Veterinary

Centre. It is an old and ornate cabinet, with beautiful curved glass sides, and came from the old surgery, at 23 Kirkgate, where Donald Sinclair (Siegfried Farnon) and Alf Wight (James Herriot) worked for all of their famous working lives. According to Pete and Tim, my partners at Skeldale, who had the pleasure of working with these two, this cabinet housed the latest medicines and shampoos, tonics and injections, and took pride of place in the waiting room. To peruse it now is like looking through a veterinary museum and, on a difficult day when I need reminding of the great heritage of our practice, I often spend a few minutes peering through its curved sides at the veterinary miscellany that sits on its shelves.

On the top shelf is an array of silver-coloured examination equipment, which would not look out of place in a museum of medieval torture: castrating tools that look barbaric to our modern eyes, a silver speculum with a spout (goodness knows what the spout was used for) and a fantastic thermocautery machine which I can remember using myself when I first arrived at Thirsk. It was affectionately referred to as 'Ronald' and in times of haemostatic crisis, when blood is leaking everywhere during an operation, a cry of 'fetch Ronald!' would instantly bring assistance running from all over the building. The machine consists of a thin metal probe or loop attached to a handpiece with a trigger. It is plugged into the mains and, when the trigger is depressed, a current flows through the metal probe to heat it up. It can then be used to cauterize, and thereby seal, bleeding vessels. This model was identical in design to a ray gun from a 1970s science fiction film, hence its pet name 'Ronald Raygun', and its comedy moniker often dispersed the anxiety that arose midway through an operation when leaking blood vessels could not be staunched. Sadly, it eventually became evident that, although Ronald was highly effective, he was a health and safety hazard, so he was put into retirement. His more youthful replacement was smaller, more nimble, easier to handle and not quite so gun-like but, in memory of his predecessor, was quickly christened 'Ronaldinho', a name which is still used today.

On the middle shelves of this cabinet are bottles of medicine. Many have labels handwritten by Mr Sinclair himself. One label features a picture of a cow, and reads:

OXYGAS

(registered title)

UDDER ILL

CHILL-IN-THE-BAG

MILK FEVER

Fever and Trembling in Sheep, Stomach Staggers

Its uses, method of administration and dosage seem obscure.

Another bottle has clearer instructions and it seems miraculous the range of conditions and number of species that could be cured with just one single tonic:

Tippers

THE BEST DRINK FOR ALL ANIMALS

'VITALIS'

For the treatment and relief of

CHILL, CATARRH, FEVER, COLIC, BLOWN, EXHAUSTION

This stuff sounds good! A full description of its functions can be found on the reverse of the bottle:

> Vitalis is pre-eminently adapted to *counteract* chill, correct abnormal temperature and tone up the constitution; increase the skin secretions by eliminating injurious waste products where the action of the kidneys is impaired and to dissipate internal gases.

> DIRECTIONS FOR USE. Tippers' Vitalis is to be given with cold water, linseed or beef tea.

It explains the doses for horse, Shire horse, yearling, cow, bullock, ewe, pig or calf, dogs, goats, kids and rabbits. Notably not cats. I suppose that either cats did not suffer any of the terrible conditions on the list, or they were not regarded as worthy of treatment in those days.

It goes on:

> N.B. If free perspiration is caused through the action of Vitalis, and the additional clothing, the rugs should be removed, the animal dried by hand-rubbing and comfortably re-clothed.

> CHILL – CATARRH – follow instructions under 'Flu':

> CHRONIC COUGH – THICK WIND – give doses of Vitalis twice daily and also give Tippers' Smirtung

It goes on further, to describe its uses in 'COLIC' in great and tedious detail, but concludes by advising that, if it doesn't work after three or four hours, then expert assistance is required. More complicated conditions, such as

'CONVALESCENCE FROM EXHAUSTION, DISTEMPER, FEVER, FLU, HOVEN, BLOWN, INFLAMMATION OF THE BOWELS, LAMBING AND CALVING, RED WATER and CATARRH IN GOATS',

all seem to require the marvellous 'Smirtung' as an adjunctive therapy, also made by Tippers. Sadly, I haven't found any of the Smirtung remedy; it must all have been used up.

My favourite medicine in the cabinet bears a handwritten label in Mr Sinclair's hand and, without listing the ingredients or dose, simply states on the label: 'For Stupefying Pigeons'.

But it is the bottom shelf that holds the most fascination for me. The envelope containing the five letters from Mr Norris on the subject of the origins of BSE still rests on a large tub, if not to say bucket, of a greasy, dark and sticky substance called 'UDDER SALVE'. This was an iodine-based ointment that was usually used for smearing on the udders of cows suffering from mastitis. If you read the letters, you would be very wary of opening the lid of this bucket for fear of the consequences.

The first reads as follows:

Dear Sir,

For eighteen years I used cow salve to beat the pain of arthrithus in my hand successfully, several different brands. This salve I bring to you killed the pain but it made me burn all over – I think this salve was taken from sheep with a desease. I am sure this salve causes mad cow desease.

Yours,
R. Norris

A second letter quickly followed:

Dear Vets,

When Mr Goodyear himself had mad cow desease he was so DIZZY he could not stand up. He had put the evil salve on several cows for a long time with his hand.

I hope you can beat this evil salve.

I milked his cows for about a week till he got organized.

Yours truly,
R. Norris

The next epistle was short but just as alarming, as the full implication of the salve on the health of cattle was becoming clear to Mr Norris:

Dear Vets,

Several cows of Mr Goodyear had mastutius, he used the <u>evil salve</u>. Mr Goodyear himself had <u>mad cow disease</u>.

Yours Truly,
R. Norris

By letter number four, Mr Norris' frustration was becoming evident; the vets were not pursuing his hypothesis with adequate vigour or enthusiasm.

Dear VETS,

I am still trying to get you to investigate the salve, which I believe causes mad cow desease. Most of the cows will be milk cows and if they were <u>in-calf</u> the calfs too could be affected. I believe the desease is slow acting. My brother goes to the lav every morning then he washes his bum and puts salve on. I think this salve is the deseased salve for the doctor told my brother he had lost the balance in his ears but I think he has mad cow desease.

R. Norris

P.S. This is my brother's daily routine.

The final note (I cannot find any further ones), is much more brief but now alludes to the dangers of this salve in other animals:

> Dear VET,
>
> I brought you the <u>evil salve</u>. What does it do to mares and foals?
>
> Yours truly,
> R. Norris

6

Monty Python

In the early days of 'Sinclair and Wight', the practice predominantly dealt with farm animals – cattle, sheep, pigs and horses. Horses were very much regarded as working animals, and were often integral to the functioning of a farm.

Many people, too, had a pig at the bottom of the garden, providing an easy supply of bacon and ham, and acting as the 1940s equivalent of a recycling bin. Dogs and cats, referred to as 'small animals' in veterinary parlance, were far fewer. Dogs were almost always working farm dogs. Cats, as the Tippers' Vitalis medicine bottle suggested, were not held in high regard. Even their potential role in rodent control was often filled by the wily Jack Russell terrier.

By the time I started work in Thirsk, the balance of work was approximately fifty-fifty. Half our time was spent seeing farm animals and horses, and the other half with small animals. While many hours were spent in the cold rain, trimming the feet of a lame cow, treating a pen of calves with pneumonia or grappling a downer cow in a muddy collecting yard, a similar amount of effort went into small animal work back at the practice. A typical day, if there ever were such a thing, would start with a couple of consultations. These were often animals that had been ill during the night, so their owners would need to bring them in before they went to work. There would usually be a case of vomiting and diarrhoea, the inside of the kitchen having been redecorated during the night (only yesterday did I see a rather handsome Doberman who had apparently 'splattered the radiator'), or these morning slots could be filled by rechecking a cat with a high temperature or blood testing a dog with diabetes, whose blood sugar levels needed to be stabilized.

After the initial half hour or so of organized chaos (it was never actual chaos, but often it felt like it), all the vets would congregate around the day book. This was where the visits for the day were written down. Some were prearranged and regular, for example 'routine visits' for dairy farms, where batches of cows were regularly checked for pregnancy. It is important that dairy cows are quickly back in calf, since this ensures a steady milk supply, so any problems must be picked up early, by regular veterinary attention. There was often a colt to castrate – a simple job if everything went according to plan, but a nightmare if things did not go smoothly. These needed some planning because two vets were required. On top of these arranged visits, emergency (and not such emergency) calls would be added to the list as the day wore on.

So every morning we would gather around the book and jobs would be assigned. As a junior vet, this was a pretty straightforward process. Typically my initials went next to all the rubbish jobs, such was the hierarchy of veterinary practice. We would also try to create a round of calls, incorporating anything from three to ten jobs all in a convenient loop, to maximize efficiency of time and travel. This was dictated by the geography of the calls and their urgency. In this way, every round inevitably encompassed a wide variety of work. Nowadays, we do far fewer visits, as there are far fewer farms, so rounds tend to be allocated according to a particular vet's area of expertise or experience, rather than down to geography.

Back then, however, it was immensely satisfying to complete a round of half a dozen calls, and manage to return to the practice before lunchtime to help finish off the ops list, invariably by polishing a cat's teeth. The vets who had been operating during the morning would do the major operations first and dental procedures would be left until the end of the ops list. This meant that dental work was always the job that I would get to finish off when I arrived back at the practice. Cleaning the teeth of a dog or cat after spending the morning wrestling with cattle, horses, sheep or pigs was a great way to round off a busy morning of work.

For veterinary surgeons who weren't out on visits, the morning's work consisted of operations, x-rays, ultrasound scanning, blood tests and so on. The practice had a busy surgical caseload, including a large number of routine neutering procedures for several local dog and cat rehoming charities (Alf Wight was instrumental in setting up one local charity based in the nearby village of Catton). Males were castrated and females spayed. Castration is relatively quick and non-invasive, but a spay is a more complex surgical procedure, involving the removal of the uterus and both ovaries. Both have considerable health benefits for the animal and, crucially for rescue charities, remove the risk of unwanted pregnancies.

Some days we would have as many as eight of these routine neutering procedures, and it could feel as if the sole purpose of a vet was to remove the gonads from our patients. It was, however, a great way to develop good surgical skills and I quickly became a confident surgeon.

The afternoon began with an open surgery from two until three and then again from five until six. Pet owners could just turn up with their sick pets during these times, without prior booking. Nowadays most veterinary surgeries operate an appointment system, where slots are booked in advance by telephone. While we now offer this system throughout the morning, we still like open surgeries and find they work well for us. The downside is that they are unpredictable and can be very busy, but there are many benefits. We have three or four vets all consulting at the same time so the workload is equally shared. If one vet gets delayed because of a complicated case, then another, with a series of more straightforward jobs, will catch up. It also allows clients to see whichever vet they want to see, most days of the week. This allows for great case continuity, which is good for the patient and client as well as the vet. It is always satisfying to follow a case through from beginning to end. Furthermore, since there are several of us consulting together, it is easy to get a second opinion from a colleague on a complicated case. Even if it is just 'Peter, can you have a quick look at this cat's eye' or 'Tim, could you palpate this dog's abdomen', it is very helpful, particularly when we have newly graduated vets working with us, because good support at an early stage of your career is incredibly important.

The atmosphere in a busy waiting room is usually bustling and vibrant, and there is usually lots of chat about the animals, how they are progressing or why their bandage is so big. It would be nice, one day if we weren't so busy, to sit in the waiting room as a 'fly on the wall' and listen to these conversations.

When afternoon surgery has finished, we usually have a couple of calls to do, or maybe an urgent operation that came through afternoon surgery. These can range from simple things like a grass seed in an ear, to exploratory surgery on a dog's abdomen. It is also a time when we try to catch up on paperwork or maybe even have a chat about practice planning or management issues. Before long, though, it is time for evening surgery, which is often the busiest part of the day. It always amuses me when I return to the practice just before five, after my afternoon visits, that so many cars are leaving the nearby workplaces to go home for the day. They must be really fit, I think, with all that free time to go to the gym or go running or cycling. Imagine how tidy their gardens must be with all that extra time in a day!

As you can see, then, our days are busy and unpredictable. One particular day, however, soon after I had started in Thirsk, was more impossible to predict than any other.

I had been out on visits all morning, and had returned to the surgery prior to heading home, via the bakers, for lunch. A call came in, and I could hear by the tone of the receptionist's voice that it was something unusual. The words 'RSPCA inspector' were mentioned followed by lots of 'okays' and then the phrase that always quickens the pulse (or makes your heart sink, if an RSPCA inspector is involved): 'I'll get someone out straight away.' As I glanced around to see my colleagues all heading out of the door with great haste, I knew this call was mine. I looked at Cathy, who had taken the message. 'You are not going to believe this, Julian … ' she said and described the situation.

The RSPCA had been called to a house, its owners having been away on holiday for a week. The neighbours were concerned because these folks had pets. There were rabbits in a hutch in the garden and some other animals in the house, which hadn't been fed or attended to for the whole week. My job, at the request of the RSPCA, was to check the animals and ascertain the state of their health. The next step, for the RSPCA, would be to establish whether cruelty had occurred. These cases can be challenging and, as the overseeing veterinary surgeon, we have to tread a delicate path, because situations are seldom quite as clear-cut as they first appear. However, for me the case had an added complication. One of the animals that had been left home alone was a Burmese python. My experience with reptiles was (and actually still is) rather limited. The 'Exotics' lectures at university were considered by many as 'semi-optional' and I am fairly sure I took the opportunity, when these lectures were scheduled, to get out on my mountain bike. On top of this, I have a dread of snakes. Snakes are, in fact, the only animal of which I am nervous, so I was not looking forward to this call, especially since this one was, apparently, huge. It would have been a challenging enough visit, had it just been the rabbits to assess. The owners (who had just returned from holiday) and the neighbours would all be stressed and anxious but, in this scenario, so would the vet.

I pulled up outside the house in my car and took a deep breath. I was greeted by an RSPCA inspector, who I knew quite well. He was very fair and helpful. He was also tall and, in his uniform, looked just like Postman Pat. This did little to lighten the atmosphere for me, though. After he had briefed me on the situation, I inspected the rabbits. They appeared healthy and had a large pile of food in their clean hutch, and they didn't need much investigation. Of course, leaving any animal unattended while heading off on holiday is never to be recommended, but the rabbits were well fed and comfortable, and seemed oblivious to their owners' absence. However, the python did not look in any way as healthy as the rabbits.

The house was a small bungalow and the main bedroom was on the ground floor. To my surprise, this was the room into which I was ushered by the inspector, to meet his assistant and the rather bewildered owners. It was a strange sight. Next to the double bed was a large glass vivarium, right in the place where most of us would have a bedside table. As if this wasn't strange enough, inside the vivarium was coiled a large, black snake. Its heat lamp was not switched on, so it was dark in the glass tank, but the form and extent of the animal was ominous and unmistakable and it was not moving.

All eyes were focused on me and I needed to do something. I remembered the advice of a fellow student at vet school: 'In times of crisis, plug your stethoscope in your ears. It'll give you time to think what to do, without being able to hear anything that people are saying to you.' So that is what I did. It gave me a moment or two of calm. Well, maybe not calm, but quiet at least.

'Right, now, what's my plan?' I thought, as I stood in the tiny bedroom. I quickly realized that I should make use of the stethoscope now it was plugged into my ears. Surely that was the best way to examine the snake. It then dawned on me that I wasn't exactly sure where along the length of its body I needed to place my stethoscope to hear its heartbeat. However, as it happens I didn't quite get the chance to find out because just as I was about to plunge the stethoscope into the tank, the owner of the snake shouted: 'Wait! Be really careful, 'cos he's very dangerous with people that he doesn't know and he doesn't like being handled!'

Great, I thought. Just what I need. Not just a massive python, the largest snake I had ever seen, but also a dangerous one. I would have been frightened by a thirty-centimetre harmless grass snake. I had to reassess my plan. At that moment, two fragments of reptilian knowledge floated to the front of my brain (I must have gone to at least one of the lectures after all). The first was 'torpor', a state of deep sleep, more like a coma, that snakes can enter when they are cold (for example, when their heat lamp is turned off) and the other was that they only need to eat infrequently, so can happily last for several weeks without food. Excellent! I had a new plan. I would suggest simply re-warming the snake by turning on the lamp in the vivarium. This would reinvigorate the reptile and I would return the following week to see it happy, awake and warm and I wouldn't need to handle it at all. Hooray.

I carefully explained my new plan, and everyone seemed satisfied. As I waved goodbye, I had a comfortable feeling of having solved the problem, avoiding certain death, and having kept everyone happy.

A week later, my plan did not look quite so brilliant.

I met the inspector at the surgery and we went to the bungalow together. We were greeted warmly by the owners, and were shown into the bedroom again (still bizarre). I had no stethoscope this time as I had no intention of handling the python, especially as I now expected it to be larger than life and happily warmed up. However, this was not the scene that met me. The first thing I noticed was the rather sweet but fetid smell. When I peered at the glass box, I was horrified to see that the snake was larger, but not larger than life. Its diameter was approximately twice what it had been the previous week. It also had a crusty topside where it was closest to the lamp. It was horribly bloated and was starting to cook. Oh dear. The poor snake. It had actually been dead the previous week and, following my instructions, it had been gently warmed up over the last seven days, hastening the process of decomposition, right next to the double bed in this small house.

We took the dead snake back to the practice to perform a very smelly post mortem examination and, at the insistence of Postman Pat, to measure it. I felt very guilty that I had subjected the owners to an increasingly malodorous week. I did wonder why on earth they hadn't called us back sooner!

Since then I have thought long and hard about this case and I can't help wondering if it was actually dead before they went on holiday, hence the reason for switching off the lamp. I guess I'll never know. The owners received a stern reprimand from Postman Pat, but I think the embarrassment and the stench were sufficient to teach them a lesson about animal management. One thing, though, is for certain – I will never forget that case. It hasn't done much for my wariness of snakes either. Or bungalows.

7

Up in the Night

Being 'on call' or 'on duty' can take a challenging and often tiring job to another level. Our working day is a long one and our skills of decision-making, diagnosis and communication are frequently tested. Within a ten-minute consultation, for example, we greet the owner, acquaint ourselves with the patient, take a history of the condition, carry out an examination (sometimes needing to employ all our powers of calming and soothing to avoid being scratched or bitten by an anxious or just plain angry patient), decide whether further tests are needed, make a diagnosis, decide upon a treatment plan, discuss this with the owner, prescribe the appropriate medication, arrange a checkup, and then cheerfully bid them both farewell. Repeat this twenty or thirty times, add a handful of operations, a list of calls and maybe a calving or lambing and that makes up a standard day in mixed practice.

When the day comes to an end, the phones are put through to a message handling service. They answer the calls that come in during the evening and through the night. One lucky person gets to put bleep one in his pocket. Another, slightly luckier, gets to have bleep number two. Being on call is a necessary evil for a veterinary surgeon, and puts considerable constraints upon our home lives. The first-on-call vet, with bleep number one, is paged by the message handling service as calls come in. These can be absolutely anything, from life-threatening emergencies like calvings, horses with colic, bloated cows or cats that have been run over, to people wanting to book an appointment for the following day, a guinea pig with a piece of carrot stuck in its mouth, or a dog that hasn't eaten its tea. The vet who is second-on-call is there to help out if two emergencies arise at the same time (this often happens at lambing time) or if the first-on-call vet needs assistance with an operation, such as a caesarean. It is usually much quieter on second call than it is on first, although there are exceptions.

One Easter weekend, Tim was called to rescue a dog from the fast lane of the A19. The dog, subsequently christened Mac (short for Tarmac), had been hit on the road more than once, and had broken all four of his legs. So severe were his injuries that on this occasion three vets had to be called in, all to operate at the same time to repair his broken limbs. Mac went on to make a full recovery and was adopted by our practice cleaner, Julie, who owns a smallholding in Thirsk. I would see Mac lolloping around with the hens whenever I called at Julie's to help lamb her sheep or vaccinate her horses. A couple of his broken legs were left a bit wonky, but his recovery was spectacular, considering the terrible injuries he had sustained.

The rota is equally shared, and we all work two nights on call during the week (one on first, one on second) and approximately one in two weekends. A weekend on duty can sometimes feel equivalent to a full week of work if it is busy, and we are straight back into the breach on Monday morning. One summer, I remember working four weekends in a row, a first, then a second, then another first followed by another second. It was thirty-three days of work without a day off.

Friday night marks the beginning of a weekend on call. I love coming down Sutton Bank on the way back from the first visits of the evening. If the weather is clear the view stretches from Swaledale in the north, through Wensleydale and Nidderdale with Wharfedale behind, and on into the far distance, where you can see Emley Moor mast in the heart of the West Yorkshire Pennines. Looking down the Vale of York, it is sometimes even possible to see the tower of York Minster. Our patch, at least for farm animal and equine work, is spread over a radius of about 15 miles, and it always feels a privilege to be looking after all the animals in this beautiful landscape. It tempers the anxiety one feels when wondering what the rest of the weekend might have in store. If an evening call takes me in the opposite direction, towards the Vale of York, my return journey brings me back through the middle of town, where there is the bustle and excitement of busy pubs and restaurants, full of folks relaxing after their week of work. There is no relaxation for the vet on call though.

Sometimes, as a young assistant on call on a Friday night, I would stop on my way through town for fish and chips. There are some excellent fish and chip shops in Thirsk, perfect for a quick and filling tea for a hungry young vet. On one occasion I was returning, tired and hungry, from a calving. The shop was fairly full, but the queue seemed to evaporate when I walked in, and I could not understand why the waiting customers had fallen silent. It was only when I got back home to tuck in that I realized I had blood all over my forehead and cheeks.

I looked like some kind of mass murderer. It was apparently a good way of jumping the queue. I should try the same trick in Tesco.

It is often the case that difficult jobs are the most rewarding, and some of the most memorable times while working as a veterinary surgeon have been associated with being on call. Nowadays, many practices, particularly those dealing only with small animals, especially in urban areas, do not undertake their own out-of-hours work, but instead employ the services of an emergency clinic. I can't help feeling that, while the vets undoubtedly have an easier and more balanced life, they are missing out on a lot of the excitement, and the biggest challenges. Many young veterinary surgeons now choose jobs where there is no out-of-hours work. This means they are less likely to be exposed to some of the most rewarding cases that veterinary medicine has to throw at us.

Two of my favourite patients – Fred and Poppy Martin, both Great Danes – came to our practice directly as a result of their previous vets handing their out-of-hours provision over to an emergency centre. The Martins were adamant that they wanted the same vets to treat their dogs at midnight as at 9.30 in the morning, so, based on a personal recommendation, they decided to come to our practice. They travel from a great distance to see us. Being Great Danes, both dogs are prone to the most serious, challenging and life-threatening emergency that we see in our job: gastric dilatation and volvulus (GDV). This is a dramatic and rapidly developing condition, whereby the stomach blows up with gas and then twists, causing catastrophic effects on the body. If it is not treated within about an hour, death follows quickly.

Both dogs have had the misfortune to suffer from a GDV,

so their owners are very alert to subtle changes that might indicate the development of the condition. Since they have a journey of about forty-five minutes to get to the surgery, they usually jump into the car and set off at the first sign of any possible problem, phoning the practice en route. On one occasion, in the middle of the night, their speeding Land Rover, with a bloated dog on the back seat, was pulled over by the police, on the A1 somewhere north of Thirsk. After a brief discussion, it transpired that the policeman knew the practice, and indeed me, the vet on call, very well. In his pre-uniform days he used to keep cattle and pigs at a farm near Thirsk. Rather than a reprimand (or worse) for the driver, he gave them a high-speed police escort directly to the surgery! There followed three hours of emergency surgery to decompress and untwist Fred's stomach, sew it back into place, and to remove his spleen, which had been badly and irreversibly damaged because the torsion had cut off its blood supply. It was a difficult and exhausting night's work, but incredibly rewarding, and one of those occasions that ultimately makes you a better vet. I still see Fred regularly. He now has a serious heart condition called dilated cardiomyopathy. The textbooks tell me he should have been dead two years ago, but Fred stubbornly refuses to follow the rules. When he comes for his monthly checkups, I always think of his night-time blue light trip, which undoubtedly saved his life.

There is an amazing variation in our on-call work. It will oscillate wildly between a genuinely life-threatening emergency, such as Fred or a horse with colic, to the dog that I saw last night at midnight, who had a sore tail. The yellow Labrador came running into the practice, vigorously wagging the aforementioned tail with great enthusiasm. It was not quite the emergency that had been portrayed down the telephone, and a dose of pain relief was all that was required. I always wonder if the same kind of thing happens in hospital casualty departments. It is amazing how different the perception of an emergency can be from one person to the next.

It is not just the night and weekend duties that get in the way of a 'normal' life. Holiday periods like Christmas, New Year and Easter are often disrupted too. Luckily for me, my wife is also a veterinary surgeon, so understands perfectly the pressures of on-call life (although her practice uses an emergency out-of-hours service), and my kids are used to it and accept it as standard. My youngest son, Archie, is perfectly *au fait* with terminology like 'on second', which means a trip to the local skate park is feasible, but a mountain bike ride is not. It means I can take him to swim training but not to a gala. For Jack, who is older, 'first call' means I can drop him off at his tennis match in Ripon, but he might need to wait around afterwards, or get a lift home with friends. They accept it as a minor inconvenience but mercifully have never held it against me. It is, after all, what they have grown up with. For the rest of my relatives, it is more difficult. I am frequently unable to attend family Christmas parties or significant birthdays, or I just turn up, say a brief 'hello' then make a hasty getaway, because I have asked a colleague to stand in for me for an hour or so.

Over Christmas and New Year we share out the on-call duties so everyone gets some time off. We always try to finish early on Christmas Eve, which feels like a festive treat. We never get away, however, without the traditional Christmas Eve call to attend an animal up in Hawnby, at the farm furthest away from the surgery. Invariably, they find a lame bull, a cow off colour or a couple of calves that are 'not quite right'. It takes half an hour to get there in good weather, but much longer if there is snow on the ground, so whoever goes up there is late home for their mince pies.

I can remember my first Christmas as a vet. I was working on the day itself, so planned to visit my family in Castleford on Christmas Eve. My mum was going to make Christmas dinner and we were going to exchange presents, as if it was Christmas Day. I managed to avoid the Hawnby call and headed fifty minutes down the A1, for Christmas dinner a day early. It was a lovely evening, and actually a perfect time to eat a big dinner, as I had been working all day. I also remember the Christmas present I was given by my parents – my first-ever mobile phone. Before the widespread use of mobile phones, we had to stop at a telephone box if our beeper went off, so this very heavy device, with a battery life of about thirty minutes, was transforming.

I stayed in Castleford overnight and got up early on Christmas morning to drive back to Thirsk. On days like these, the duty vets usually meet up at the surgery to hand over beepers, check the inpatients and exchange case notes. We would wryly offer each other the season's greetings, in the knowledge that Christmas might not be quite as festive as it could be. During one Christmas holiday, a local farmer had a complete disaster when he discovered that the bull he had used on all his cows had produced calves too enormous to be delivered on their own. Almost every one required veterinary attention, so when we exchanged our beepers, we would compare the number of calvings or caesareans we had performed at his farm, Vicar's Moor, over the last twenty-four or forty-eight hours, and how huge the calves had been. Of course, we always tried to describe a more fantastical scenario than our colleagues.

On this, my first Christmas morning as a veterinary surgeon, I had a not-too-festive visit at 8.30 a.m. to see a very poorly calf, suffering from severe pneumonia. The farm was beset by a variety of problems, and we were frequent visitors. I can remember the sharp December air, the damp straw and the poor little calf with a raging temperature of 107 degrees Fahrenheit, as clearly as yesterday. I also remember the farmer making not a single reference to it being Christmas day at all! No 'Merry Christmas', no 'Sorry to have to get you out today', not a thing.

I returned home for a coffee and was about to sit down with a mince pie when my beeper was in action again. This time it was a cat that was 'not quite right'.

'Well, she's sitting under the piano. Can you come and look at her?'

House visits are generally much more challenging than examinations at the surgery. It is hard to keep the animal in a suitable position to be examined, the light is often poor, the television is invariably blaring, and we have a more limited selection of equipment and medication than is available at the surgery. We prefer, therefore, to see patients at the practice. However, in this case the cat was sitting under the piano and apparently could not be caught. Also (and probably more to the point), since the pre-dinner sherry had been broached in the middle of the morning, the cat's owners were in no fit state to transport it in a car.

I had an idea what would follow, and I was right. I spent forty-five minutes crawling around on the floor of the Christmassy house, trying to catch the cat that had made a miraculous recovery as soon as this strange man, smelling vaguely of surgical spirit, had appeared.

I was unable to examine it in much detail. I managed to administer a precautionary injection and suggested that they bring the cat to the surgery for a checkup after the holiday. Again, there was no 'Sorry to disturb you', not even a 'Merry Christmas' and certainly no mince pie! I wasn't particularly bothered by this, just somewhat surprised by the general lack of festive cheer.

Back home again, I put the kettle on and at last considered the possibility of that mince pie. But no, the bleeper went again. This time it was an elderly gentleman, whom I knew to be more poorly than his little dog. The terrier had terrible respiratory disease. We went out regularly to administer extra medication because his owner, Mr Moss, also had severe emphysema and needed to be attached to an oxygen machine for long periods. I knew that Mr Moss would be by himself today, as always. Since I had not yet eaten my mince pies, I decided to take them with me to his house to share, and we sat together, accompanied by the hissing of the oxygen machine, eating mince pies, while I injected his dog with steroids. It was not quite the Christmas day I had expected, but I was glad Mr Moss had not had to spend it alone. It was the most important thing I had done that day, and it had nothing to do with veterinary medicine.

———

Usually, if we work Christmas, we don't work New Year and vice versa. It is always a busy time, as winter lambing and calving are both in full swing and people are out and about on their horses, and with their dogs. Interestingly, though, wishes of 'Happy New Year' are frequent when we are called out during this part of the festive season.

The first call of the year, I feel, sometimes sets the tone for the rest of the year ahead. Four years ago I got a call at 2 a.m. on 1 January from a local farmer. He was in a terrible tizz; he had a cow with her 'calf bed out'. This condition is technically called a uterine prolapse. It happens shortly after calving, particularly if the calf was big, or the delivery difficult. The whole uterus is pushed out, and turns completely inside out, just like a sock that has been pulled off a foot in a hurry. These cases are a major emergency, because the inverted uterus quickly gets covered in straw and other debris and can even be trodden on by the cow. Some cows remain lying down, so the uterus is less likely to be trodden on, but gets very dirty, while others wander around with an organ as big and as heavy as a sack of potatoes hanging out of their back end. It is extremely physical work to replace the swollen and often damaged uterus, and is guaranteed to leave the veterinary surgeon hot, sweating and covered in blood and dirt. An old vet called Eddie Straiton, a friend and contemporary of Alf Wight, reputedly recommended that the vet should strip off completely to perform this procedure, to save his clothes from ruin. I had no intention of following Eddie's advice on this freezing night.

When I arrived, a very worried farmer greeted me. He had clearly been enjoying the New Year celebrations earlier in the evening, and wasn't handling his cow's problem well. He was rushing around, without being much help, so I asked for a bucket of warm water, in the hope that this simple job would give him something useful to do and calm his anxiety. When he returned he recounted the horrific sight of this enormous uterus appearing and how, as soon as he saw it emerging from the cow's vulva, he had rushed inside to phone me. He had not been back to check the cow after he made the phone call, so when we arrived at the yard where she was penned, the situation was not quite as I had expected. In fact, there was a happy, healthy, normal cow licking her lovely newborn calf. Next to this calf was a huge pile of afterbirth. This is the placenta, which is passed five or ten minutes after the birth of the calf (hence its name). The inebriated farmer had seen this appearing and mistaken it for a prolapsing uterus, panicked, and phoned for help. Rather apologetically, he wished me a Happy New Year and we laughed about it. I couldn't have been more relieved. It made for a very simple first call of the year and I didn't even have to get my hands (or the rest of me) dirty.

8

Sabrina's Dead?

Skeldale was, and still is, a brilliant place for a young vet to start their veterinary career. It strikes an ideal balance, allowing clinical freedom and the chance to develop, while providing support and back-up when required. Since there are always two vets on duty, there is always someone to call upon for help or advice and, because we are based at only one site, a young vet is never left manning a branch surgery singlehandedly. We usually consult together, so we can easily ask for a second opinion from the vet in the next consulting room. Similarly, we usually have several vets operating at any one time. While one person is taking x-rays, another may be doing a dental, so help is always at hand. Furthermore, most of our farm and equine clients are within half an hour's drive of the surgery, so it is easy to ask a colleague to visit a sick cow or a lame horse to give a second opinion. I can remember, as a new graduate, doing exactly this, when I had been treating a very expensive hunter, which had been caught in barbed wire.

I went to see this beautiful horse late one November evening, not long after starting work in Thirsk. I arrived at the very grand Warlaby Hall, and then had something of a search around the enormous grounds to find the patient. It is often the case that you arrive at an emergency on a farm or at a yard to find no one there to meet you. As a young vet, you very quickly get over your embarrassment at having to poke your head into sheds and knock on random doors, or even wander into people's houses in your quest for the patient, when time is of the essence.

When I eventually found the horse, it was surrounded, as is usually the case in such emergencies, by a swarm of anxious faces with torches, and there was an atmosphere of palpable stress and worry. I assessed the situation and decided to sedate the horse so I could carry out a proper examination. It was very shocked and stood very still while I gave it the intravenous sedative combination. The poor animal had a large laceration on its back leg, just at the level of the fetlock. It had severed a major artery and lost a large flap of skin. Barbed wire and horses is a terrible, but quite common, combination. I managed to clamp and then ligate (tie off) the bleeding vessel without incident – treating back leg injuries in horses is fraught with potential danger and risk of injury to the vet from metal-shod hooves, so our main priority in these cases is to avoid being kicked in the head. All was uneventful, and the hole in the skin came together reasonably well. I applied a bandage, administered some antibiotics and the all-important anti-tetanus injection (horses are very prone to tetanus) and headed back to the surgery, to see a poorly rabbit.

Three weeks passed and the wound on the horse's leg had failed to heal as fully as I had hoped, so I asked Pete for help. Rather than simply give me instructions, he kindly said, 'I know, let's go to see it together.' Off we went, late one morning, to look at the wound. I hadn't done anything wrong. Wounds on horses' legs are just slow to heal, but that support helped my confidence, and dispelled any doubts the owner may have had over the handling of the case by a newly qualified vet.

At this time, the other equine enthusiast in the practice was my friend and colleague, David. He too was a Cambridge graduate, like Jon and me. David was a good friend of my girlfriend Anne (they were at the same college, shared a house and played violin in the university orchestra together) and he was the one who had introduced me to the practice. He is a passionate veterinary surgeon with a huge appetite for knowledge and always strives for a perfect diagnosis and exemplary treatment. This makes him an excellent vet, and he is now a clinician at Glasgow veterinary school, but his academic approach was not always perfectly suited to what was, at that time, a basic and often rugged mixed practice. He was perfectly happy investigating a complex case, maybe of a horse which was losing weight or a dog whose blood count was slightly too low. No stone would be left unturned in his quest for the solution to his patients' problems. He was very well liked, and some of our older clients still talk fondly of his compassionate manner. A few of the more gruff farmers, however, were not so taken by his fastidious methods and would refuse to have him calve their cows or examine their pneumonic bulls. How wrong this minority was, because he invariably got everything right.

David was a brilliant vet and a delight to work with, although he could be frustrating for the partners. He had very little awareness of good financial management, and also had a terrible sense of direction.

He would often head off on a visit, get hopelessly lost, and be gone from the practice all day. One Christmas Day, Pete had invited David, who was on call, to join his family for Christmas lunch. David had taken his violin to play carols before and after dinner, but arrived well into the pudding course, having spent hours calling at every house in the villages of Great and Little Thirkleby, rather than the village of Thirlby, where Pete actually lived.

David was a great storyteller, too, and his anecdotes could rival even Jim Wight's stories (as Herriot's son, Jim is a master of the art of telling a tale). His description of the time he went to perform a semen test on a miniature dachshund was hilarious. David, like me, had been taught how to do this by the famous Dr Jackson, so he was well qualified to perform the task. Instead of using an examination table, as we had been shown, David performed the procedure on the elderly lady's kitchen table. As if this wasn't peculiar enough, he amusingly recounted how he kept the microscope slides warm (so he could analyse the sperm at the correct temperature) by placing them on the grill of the oven!

During the year I worked with David at Thirsk, he taught me an awful lot. Not necessarily factually, but more about the importance of being thorough and meticulous.

Just before my first Christmas at Skeldale, David had been presented with an injured owl. It had been found nearby the surgery and brought in by a member of the public. He had spent a full morning meticulously repairing its broken wing, ingeniously using hypodermic needles as makeshift bone pins. As hypodermic needles are hollow and therefore lightweight, they were perfect for repairing the fractured bones of a bird.

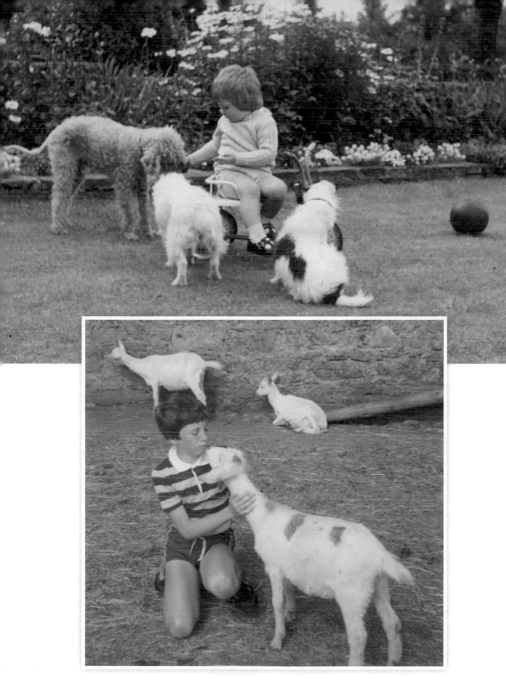

Even as a young boy I loved being surrounded by animals.

Top: Here I am at my grandparents' house with Judy, the Bedlington, and Paddy and Sue, the Jack Russells.

Above: On a family holiday in Wales I never missed a chance to be with animals, in this case a goat.

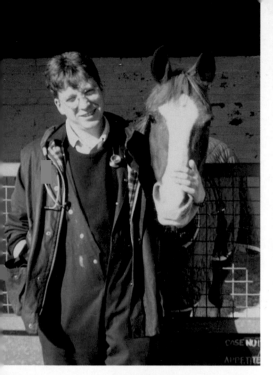

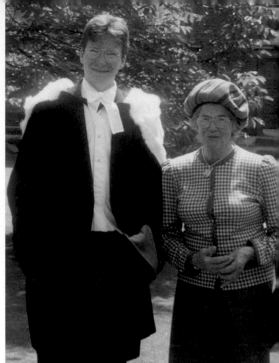

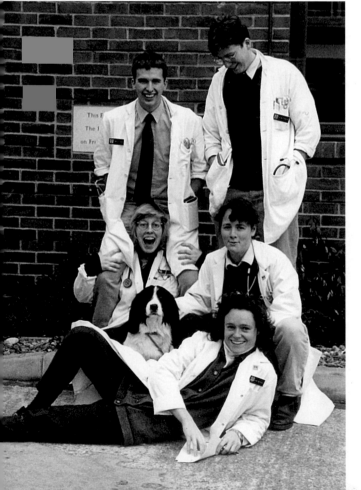

Above left: While at vet school we had opportunities to visit other universities and this picture is at Leahurst, the equine unit of Liverpool's vet school.

Above: My Gran and me on my graduation day at Pembroke. Gran was a true inspiration to me and spent much of her life with animals. We were very close during the early part of my life.

Left: This is my clinical group at vet school. We worked hard and played hard – from top left, Ben, me, Jenny, Cath and Claire.

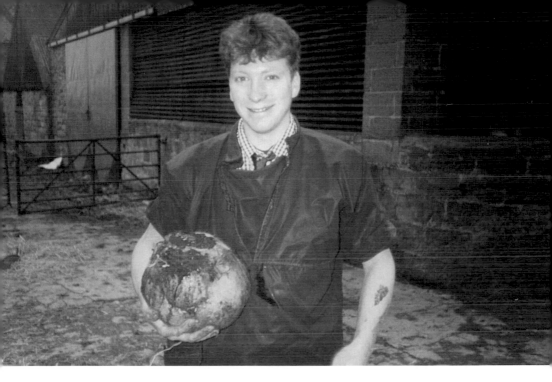

Above: Soon after starting work at Skeldale, my colleague Tim and I removed this massive lump from the neck of a heifer. It was bigger than a football.

Below: A young Paddy and me relaxing on the sofa. He was just like a teddy bear!

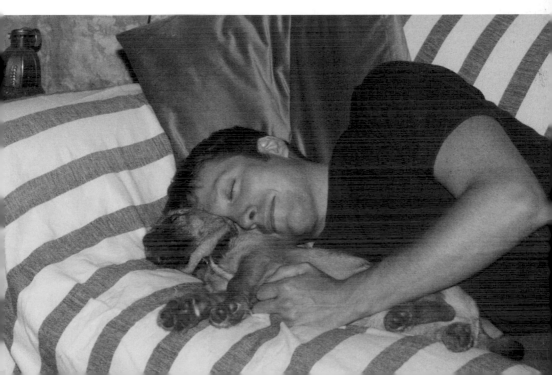

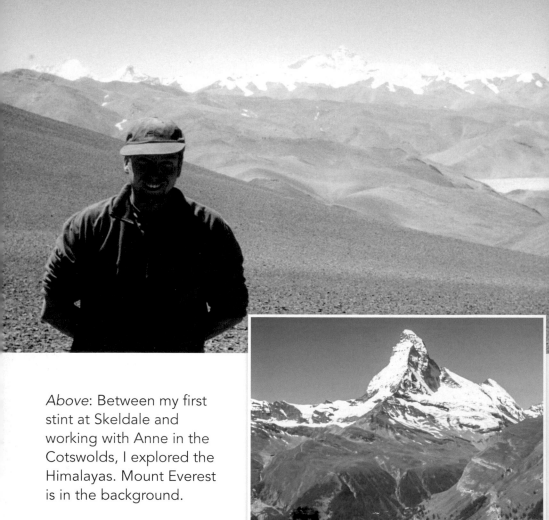

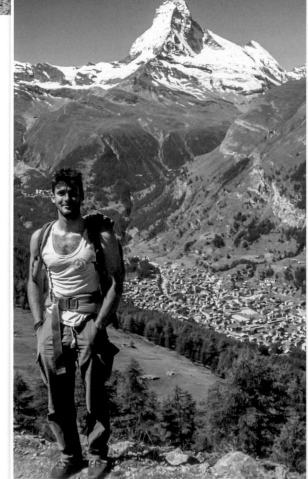

Above: Between my first stint at Skeldale and working with Anne in the Cotswolds, I explored the Himalayas. Mount Everest is in the background.

Right: Dave Payne in the Swiss Alps, with the Matterhorn behind, where disaster would strike three weeks later.

Far right: Anne and me on our wedding day, 21 October 2000. It was a great day in Hampshire.

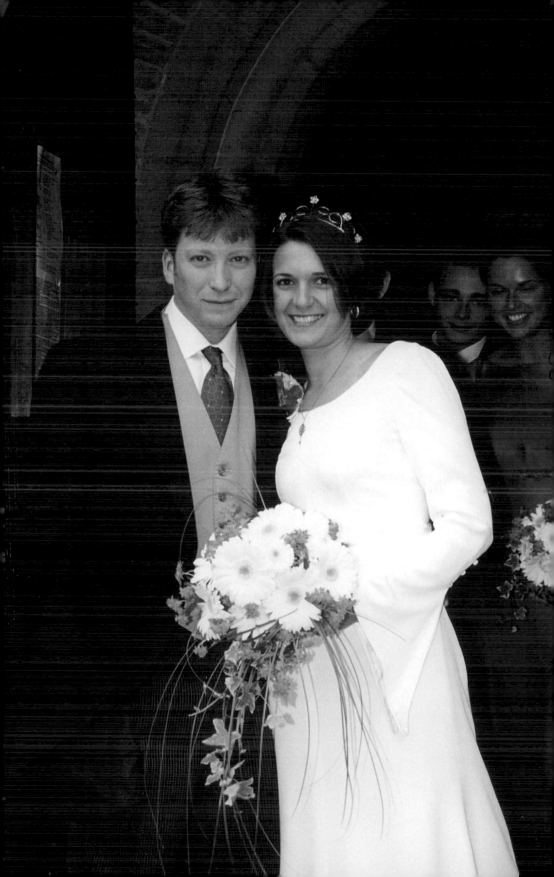

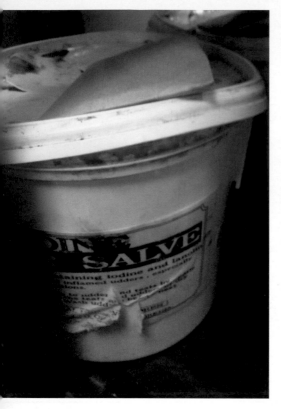

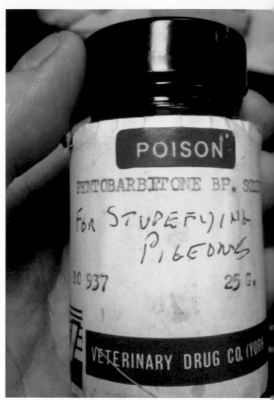

The Evil Salve, medicine for stupefying pigeons and other concoctions in the old cabinet upstairs at our practice in Thirsk.

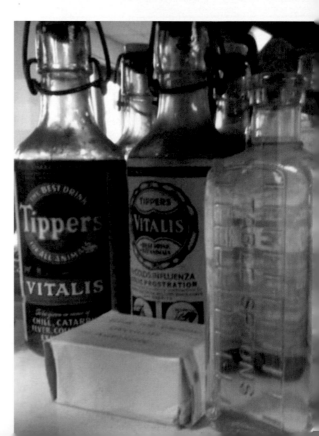

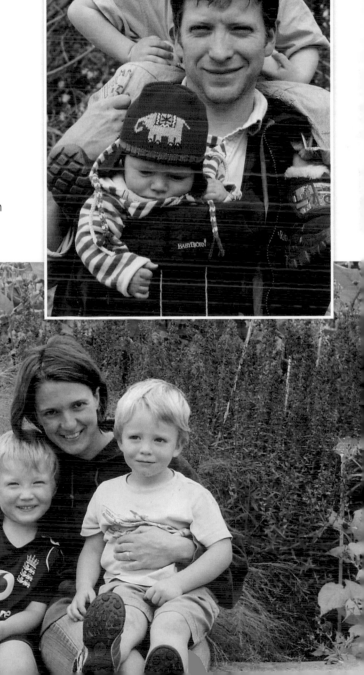

Right: Feeling the weight of two growing boys. Jack took his tennis balls everywhere with him and Archie looks pensive.

Below: Anne, Jack and Archie on a summer day at Harlow Carr Gardens in Harrogate.

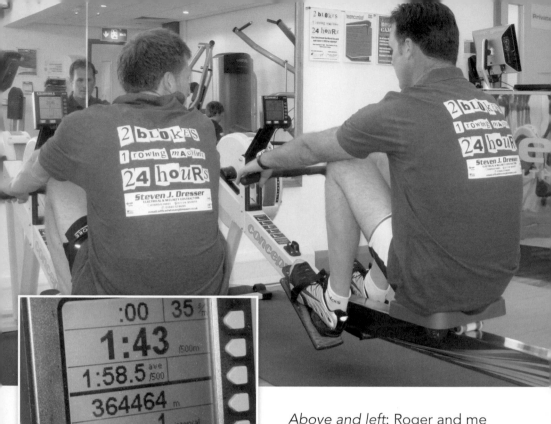

Above and left: Roger and me training for our attempt at the world record for 24-hour rowing as a tandem on the Concept 2 indoor rowing machine. The screen on the left shows our distance, a new world record and an impressive average split of 1.58.5 for each 500m.

Left: Another proud moment: representing Team GB, for my age group, in the European Middle-Distance Triathlon championships in Paguera, Mallorca, in 2014.

The owl had been with us for over a week, recuperating from its operation. I had been helping David during this time and we had both become attached to our feathery patient. On Christmas Eve, after the rest of the practice staff had gone home, we decided the time was right to release the bird back to its natural habitat. Its wing looked strong and although the owl did not know it was Christmas, it seemed appropriate to let him go home on this day. We carefully carried him outside, towards the neighbouring fields, and held him aloft. He stretched his wings and we felt confident that he would fly unhindered. He looked all around and I gently flicked him into the air. To our delight, he flew off, into the washed out, wintery sunshine and headed straight to a large oak tree just between the practice and the fields. He had flown effortlessly and it was a joy to see him going so well, justifying of all our efforts.

Sadly, our joy was only momentary. Our owl landed on a large, high branch of the oak tree, but misjudged his landing and tumbled, bouncing off lower branches until he fell, splat onto the road. As we rushed towards the road to retrieve him and take him back into the clinic, a lorry thundered past, and to our horror, went straight over him, leaving a flurry of feathers where the owl once was. We were devastated. It was not a good start to Christmas for any of us, especially not the owl.

After about a year, David moved on, into academia. His replacement was another equine enthusiast called Ben. Jon, Ben and I had a lot in common and we worked superbly as a team. It was simply a joy to wake up in the morning and go into work. We were having so much fun, it didn't really seem like work at all. Ben had a brilliant manner with clients and was an eloquent orator. It soon became clear that client communication was one of his great talents. He would explain conditions and treatments in minute detail, and capture the imagination of the enthralled owners with his florid descriptions. Mostly they were based on fact, but sometimes I was not so sure. His main recommendation for almost any abdominal condition in dogs was the feeding of 'moist green vegetables'.

The art of client communication, be it face to face in a consultation or over the telephone, is a great skill to master and is a crucial part of veterinary practice. Ben was very adept, but it was a skill that I was slower to perfect.

One of my worst errors in this department is forever etched on my mind. In my penultimate year at Cambridge, I was offered a four-week externship at the illustrious Veterinary Hospital, University of Pennsylvania (or VHUP for short) in the USA. It was one of the leading centres of veterinary excellence and it was an amazing opportunity. I spent two weeks in the emergency department and two weeks in the medicine department.

We worked a fourteen-hour shift, either days or nights, and each shift would comprise twelve hours in the clinic followed by two hours of tutorials and case discussions. Afterwards we would eat a massive pizza and then sleep, wake up, drink an enormous vat of coffee and do the same again. I did this non-stop for a month and learnt a huge amount. It was very exciting in the emergency department, and we were faced with conditions that would rarely be seen in a rural practice in England. 'High-Rise Cats', for instance, were cats that had accidentally fallen from windows in high-rise apartment blocks, and we saw GSWs (gunshot wounds) to dogs that had been caught up in drive-by shootings.

On the medical wards we had responsibility for complicated cases that would be hospitalized for long periods. The Americans did not do things by halves, and we were required to take blood samples four times daily to monitor for subtle changes in our patients. I was never completely sure that this was strictly necessary or indeed helpful – there were stories of dogs who had developed anaemia from having had too many blood samples taken – but it was certainly thorough, and a fantastic learning experience.

I had one particularly memorable patient. She was a large and lovely Doberman called Sabrina. Her blood count was peculiar and it was postulated that this had been caused by an obscure reaction to some medication that had been prescribed by a different vet. I was not fully convinced by this explanation of her illness, but the supportive treatment seemed to be working and she was progressing well, despite my six-hourly blood sampling.

I was in the habit of telephoning the owners of all my patients every evening, to give an update on their progress before I left to get my obligatory pizza for tea. Sabrina's owners were very worried about their beloved dog, so I would always phone them last, so I had plenty of time to discuss things in detail. On this occasion, towards the end of Sabrina's stay in the hospital, I called her owners to give a final update before they came to collect her the following day.

'Oh hello, is that … ' I said, and then completely forgot the chap's surname. I panicked and quickly changed tack. 'Hello,' I said in my obviously obscure Not-Just-English-But-Yorkshire accent, 'Is that Sabrina's dad?'

I thought this had got me out of the hole. But no! My unfamiliar accent had been misunderstood.

'OH MY GOD!' he screamed. It might have been Woody Allen by the frenzy and desperation in his voice.

'I'LL GET MY WIFE … HONEY, SABRINA'S *DEAD!*'

I was mortified, and it took me a long time to convince them that she was not at all dead, but very much alive and ready to go home the following day.

The next day, when Sabrina was discharged, fit, well and alive, I was presented with a baseball cap from the guy's favourite team, so I think I was forgiven. In my final 'debrief', the senior clinician at VHUP offered me an internship for my first job after graduating, so I guess I hadn't messed up too badly. I seriously considered the offer, but in the end I couldn't imagine not being in Yorkshire. I often wonder how different my life would have been had I taken up that offer.

Ben was not only much better at client communication than I was, but he was enormous fun to work with. We had a half-day each week, to make up for our long hours, and Ben and I both had ours on a Thursday afternoon. This suited me because my night on first-call was a Wednesday, so if I'd had a busy night, I knew I only had four hours of work before I could go home. We would often head to the hills on our mountain bikes. Our favourite route took us around the edge of the Hambleton Hills, Boltby Forest and the moors around Hawnby and Snilesworth. We would sometimes see farmers that we knew, as they went about their business on tractors, although as we were clad in bright helmets and colourful Lycra, they never seemed to recognize us! The route led us to a superb descent through a narrow gully of rhododendrons, which ended up in the pretty little village of Kepwick. It was fast, rocky and dangerous and could only rarely be achieved without putting a foot down. I did the same route three weeks ago with my oldest son, Jack. It is still fast, steep and dangerous, but now, nearly twenty years later, the rhododendron bushes have grown to completely enclose the gully. Rather than being open-topped, it is now a 400-metre-long leafy tunnel and in parts it is impossible to see the sky above.

Thursday afternoon rides would sometimes take us further afield. In winter, we had just enough time to drive into the middle of the North York Moors, and in summer I could drive to the Lake District, cycle up Helvellyn and return in time for a couple of quick pints in the Blacksmith's Arms in the middle of town. This was our usual watering hole. Thirsk has a heritage as a coaching town. Before the railway arrived, travel up and down the country was by stagecoach, so the town was well supplied with pubs and inns. In the 1990s, we could choose one of about fifteen pubs within a stone's throw of the market square. When Jim and Pete were at a similar stage in their careers, there were over twenty. Half a pint in each was a standard Saturday night challenge.

On our first New Year here, we invited loads of vet friends from university up to Thirsk for a New Year's Eve celebration. After a hastily prepared Mexican meal at home, we walked to the market square to sample the pubs, and Jon and I were proud to show off our home town.

Thirsk looks lovely at Christmas, with simple lights strung all around the large, cobbled square, with its clock tower at the centre, next to the massive iron bull ring set into cobbles, from the days when livestock were traded regularly here.

Now, I had enjoyed many New Year's Eve parties in other

North Yorkshire towns, notably in nearby Knaresborough, Ripon and Helmsley. In these places, just before midnight, everyone leaves the pubs to collect around the cross or the clock in the town square, and await the chimes that signify the old year passing and the New Year arriving. There is a huge communal celebration and it is all very festive. So, at about half past eleven, the group of about twenty of us wandered outside to get a good spot in the middle. We waited patiently with three policemen who were there in case of trouble later. As I chatted with the bobbies, and the time crept closer to midnight, I couldn't help but notice that we were still standing by ourselves, with no throngs of revellers anywhere to be seen. This seemed odd and in complete contrast to what I was expecting. When the clock struck twelve, our group of young vets celebrated a rather muted New Year with three very sober policemen and nobody else. This had been something of a flop. We decided to go back to the pub, where clearly the people of Thirsk traditionally greeted the arrival of the New Year, but when we tried to get back into the Blacksmith's Arms, the doors had been locked, as it was past closing time. Our evening's celebrations had been brought to a premature end, and our friends who had travelled to see us and partake in Yorkshire hospitality had been sorely disappointed.

For me, the premature end to the night was something of a blessing, because I was on duty the following morning and, unlike some New Year's mornings, I can remember what happened next very clearly. I was on call from 8 a.m. that morning and I was soon clambering over the slumbering bodies of my vet friends after receiving a request to visit another dairy herd, high up above the picturesque villages, on the edge of the Hambleton hills. The herd comprised about a hundred black and white Friesian cows and the place was renowned, within the practice, for its poor organization. Disasters were frequent.

The farm was cold and windswept when I arrived, but to my surprise, the sight that met me was not too dissimilar to the one I had seen the previous evening in the Blacksmith's Arms. During the night, the cows had enjoyed their own New Year's Eve party. They had, inexplicably, broken into the feed store. 'Cake' is the concentrated form of cattle food that dairy cows are fed when they are being milked. It is high in energy and designed to fuel them to produce gallons of milk. They usually receive controlled amounts of a few kilograms twice a day at milking time. These greedy (or hungry) animals had broken down the door of the shed where the food was stored, and eaten about a month's worth of food in one evening.

When a cow eats too much cow cake, the concentrated food is rapidly fermented in the rumen – part of its four-chambered stomach – and it produces a cocktail of chemicals that creates exactly the same effect on the cow as beer does on a human. The whole herd was suffering from acidosis. I surveyed the scene. Some cows were standing around the perimeter of the field, simply staring at the hedge, as if not sure what to do or where to go. Some cows were lying down in inappropriate places, their heads lolling to one side. The odd one even had its tongue hanging out of the side of its mouth. Any animal that was trying to move around was travelling very slowly and methodically. Mostly, the moving cows were meandering in a wobbly way and occasionally one would topple over into the mud. All that was needed to complete the scene were a few party hats.

The diagnosis was easy enough, but what on earth was I going to do to treat the whole herd? It was clearly not going to be fixed by a few cups of strong tea and a round of bacon sandwiches! I could not treat a hundred cows – I didn't have sufficient drugs in my car, or even in the whole practice. Handling that many drunk animals would surely also be a silly idea – cows would be falling all over the place as they were corralled into a handling pen and this would only cause more problems. I decided to leave the mild cases as they happily stared at the hedge, and concentrated on the more serious ones – the cows lying on the concrete with their heads lolling and their tongues hanging out.

I stomach-tubed about ten animals with a mixture of tonics that was basically equivalent to twenty litres of Alka-Selzter each, and then moved on to the worst two cases. In these two I decided that the only proper thing to do was to perform a rumenotomy. This is a surgical procedure where an incision is made through the skin on the left side of the cow's abdomen and into its rumen, the largest chamber of the cow's system of compound stomachs. I emptied out the stomach contents of each of these two animals into a large bucket, then flushed them out with warm tap water. This was the bovine equivalent of having their stomachs pumped. It worked well and I am happy to say that all the cows survived that day. I returned home several hours later, smelling very badly. I clambered over the slumbering bodies of my vet friends who were suffering from their own, beer-induced, acidosis, to make my way to the shower.

My next job involved making a lot of strong tea and a few rounds of bacon sandwiches.

9

Working with the Herriot Vets

In 1996, as I was graduating, Jim Wight took the decision to scale back his work as a veterinary surgeon in order to write the biography of his father, Alf Wight. It was decided that the practice should take on a new graduate – me – to fill Jim's full-time role, while Jim continued to work at the surgery two days a week. Jim was a great enthusiast and endlessly positive. I love being around people like that, as it is a contagious attitude. He had a wealth of veterinary experience, and the stories he told were sufficient in themselves to confirm the extent of his talents as a vet. Most of his stories were of his own exploits, but he could equally regale his father's old tales, with style. He would always describe his clinical cases in elaborate detail, with great flourishes of 'fantastic' or 'amazing'. My favourite of his anecdotes was one where a farmer had phoned to request a visit for a vet to examine his bullock. Apparently it had a lump on its side 'as big as a colour television set'. The amusement to Jim and to me was the implication that a colour television set was very much bigger than the black and white variety.

When I started in Thirsk, Jim was in the practice on Mondays and Fridays. He was very popular, especially with the older and more established clients who had known him for years, and had often known his father as well. We always knew when he was in the building by the all-pervading smell of pipe smoke, as he puffed away for much of the time. At that time, the practice also provided a veterinary surgeon as inspector at the local turkey factory. The role of the vet was to oversee and uphold the health and welfare of the turkeys before slaughter. This job took up a lot of time and none of us really wanted to do it, because, important as it was, it was both unpleasant and incredibly tedious. It was a great testament to Jim that he continued to cover these monotonous shifts with the turkeys right up until he retired.

As a newly qualified vet, I was brimming with new knowledge and bursting to put it all into action. However, some supervision was often prudent, and Jim was more than happy to help. I had decided to do a tibial crest transposition on a Yorkshire terrier. This is an operation carried out to correct a slipping kneecap. The crest on the front of the tibia (the shin bone), just below the knee, is moved, to bring it better into line so that the kneecap stays in its groove, instead of popping out. It was an ambitious operation for a vet who had only been qualified for five months, and at many practices I would not have been allowed to embark upon it. This kind of thing, though, was not unusual at Skeldale. The philosophy was, and still is, to encourage our new vets to 'grasp the nettle' and get involved in more challenging surgery, obviously under close supervision, as this is the best way to learn and progress. In much the same way as Frank had supervised my first caesarean section, twelve months previously, Jim sat back, lit his pipe and prepared to talk me through the procedure.

The surgery that morning was about as tricky as it got for a new vet. It was technically challenging, fiddly and fraught with the risk of serious consequences if things went wrong. However, Jim offered calm and reassuring words of encouragement as I sawed through the top of this little terrier's tibia, having first drilled tiny holes in it so it could be carefully re-attached in the correct position. He didn't handle any of the tissues, just as Frank had avoided contact with the cow, for the very same reason, I suspect – that it would have meant foregoing his tobacco. This didn't matter, though, since his description was so clear. My only concern, as he peered over the surgical site to inspect my work, was that ash would fall into my little dog's leg and contaminate my sterile op site.

It wasn't long after I started work that Jim decided to retire completely. It was a shame that I didn't get the chance to spend more time working with him, as I am sure we would have made a great team. Jim's role as senior partner was taken over by his long-time friend and colleague Peter, with whom I still work. Peter spent much of his early career working with Jim and when the two of them get together, over a pint or a Chinese meal, or both, the anecdotes flow freely. Pete's whole existence is devoted to the practice and its wellbeing, and I sometimes fear what will happen when he is eventually worn out and has to retire!

A year after I started at Skeldale, Pete and I were invited to attend a fundraising dinner for a local animal rescue charity, the Jerry Green Foundation. It was held in the Golden Fleece in Thirsk and Fred Trueman was the guest speaker. I was a big cricket fan and loved Fred's humour. Fred himself had acquired a rescue dog from Jerry Green's, and did his best to help support the work of the charity.

The problem facing us, as usual, was that we were both on call. Pete was on first and I was on second, so theoretically he would take all the calls, and I would help out only if it got too busy or if there was a two-man job. Usually it was folly to go to a social event while on duty, but since it was local and for a charity with whom we worked closely, we felt we should both take the chance.

The meal was enjoyable and then came the after-dinner speeches, and the time for raising money. Right at this point, just as Fred was lighting his first cigar of the evening, Pete's beeper went off. It was a call to a nearby farm to see a cow, down with milk fever. As junior, I offered to go, so Pete could enjoy his coffee and the rest of the speeches. He didn't argue, and I made my apologies and scuttled off to see the cow. The farm was nearby but it took me a while to complete the job because the farmer was in the middle of milking. Most farmers milk their cows at about five in the morning and again twelve hours later at five in the evening. While this is the normal way of things, there is no special reason it has to be done so early in the morning, and Alan, who ran the herd single-handedly, was the type of bloke who liked a later start to his day. Consequently, he would still be in the milking parlour at nine in the evening, which is why he was still milking when I arrived.

Once he had finished, and I had treated the cow, I washed up and headed back to the Fleece to hear the rest of Fred's stories. The evening was nearly at a close and when I met up with Pete again he had a painful smile on his face and he confessed that he rather wished he had gone to see the cow after all. Pete is not a man who parts with his hard-earned cash readily and, after I had left, the main fundraising part of the evening began. This involved various rounds of bidding and a game where large amounts of money had to be pledged. As I said, Fred was a vigorous supporter of this animal charity and had done a good job of boosting their coffers, in large part thanks to Pete, who ended the evening with a somewhat lighter wallet than he had expected. As the archetypal Yorkshireman, an expensive evening out is never one of Pete's favourites.

———

The practice is very busy, so Pete and I rarely get time to work together on clinical cases. Obviously there are the hours that we spend on the business side of running the practice, but these are no substitute for the rewards of working on a challenging case with a colleague. However, when there is a colt to be castrated, Pete and I often join forces, as it is a procedure that we always do with two vets, one to supervise the anaesthetic and one to do the operation itself. Some veterinary surgeons castrate colts under sedation, using local anaesthesia only, which allows the horse to remain standing. This is much quicker and allows equine vets to do many in a morning. To do the procedure with the colt lying down under general anaesthesia is more involved, but we have always found it to be the best way to avoid complications. Under the right circumstances, it can be a rather relaxing hour. We try to do the operation on a clear, sunny day in spring, free from mud or flies that would contaminate the wound, and if the operation goes well and the horse recovers from its anaesthetic without event, you can imagine how pleasant it can be, sitting in a sunny field waiting for a sleepy horse to emerge from its slumbers.

While castrating a colt is very straightforward if all goes

according to plan, when things do not go smoothly, absolute disasters can occur. This is especially so if the animal has not been handled sufficiently, and is jumping and kicking while we are trying to inject it with sedatives, or if the colt has grown into a boisterous stallion. Heading out to do such a procedure is daunting.

On one particular occasion, the job had been postponed several times, because Pete and I could not get there together and the farmer, who also kept show jumpers, was insistent that it should be done by the two of us. Pete is very experienced with horses. My usual role on this farm was castrating two-year-old bulls that had been missed by previous owners – not the best job either! The farmer's insistence that only the two of us in combination should undertake the operation ought to have set some alarm bells ringing.

We arrived on the farm in thick fog. The conditions were far from ideal for castrating a colt. It was damp in the air and very muddy underfoot but the farmer was not prepared to let this chance pass, and directed us to the paddock where our patient was waiting. The sight that met us as we rounded the corner made our hearts sink into our muddy boots. The field was covered in mud rather than grass, the air was thick with fog, and through the gloom we could just make out the form of an enormous horse, with its head stretched out as if it were trying to pull away from something. In the fog, it looked like a beast from a Greek legend. It was clearly a stallion with several years of growth and strength and not at all the benign yearling we had been expecting. The beast had been caught with a lasso, which was around its neck, with a long rope attached, about 20 metres away, to a JCB digger. Usually a horse being prepared for surgery would be standing in a stable, restrained with a head collar and a short lead rope, and held confidently by its competent owner. In this case the rope was very long and the thing on the non-horse end was only capable of keeping hold of the horse by virtue of its size and solidity. It seemed an impossible task to get anywhere near this wild creature. Every time we tried to pull it closer, the horse would charge around the JCB tangling us dangerously in the rope.

To make the scene even more ridiculous, the radio in the JCB cabin had been left on, and the music drifting out of the open window was the Bob Marley song 'Three Little Birds', which blithely reassured us not to worry about a thing. We were not quite as confident as Bob was that every little thing was, in fact, gonna be all right.

Slowly but surely, however, we managed to shorten the rope so the horse was close enough to handle. The next challenge was to inject it with the right dose of sedative. If we couldn't do this, the rest of the procedure would be a disaster. I drew up a strong dose. Once this was in, the horse would become sleepy, but at this stage it was still very wild. It was also very, very cross at having been lassoed and pulled right up to the digger by its neck. I had to be accurate, quick and brave. Luckily, on this occasion, I was all three of these things. Once the horse was sedated, it was time to give the general anaesthetic, again by injection. This is another point at which things can go wrong. On one occasion I was castrating a colt with Tim. He had to climb on a stepladder to be able to inject the sedative into its vein. Despite appearing to be nicely sedated, just as I was about to give the anaesthetic, the sleepy horse looked up, bolted straight across the field and made its escape. Today, if the same thing happened, our horse would burst through the rickety fence and land in the slurry lagoon, which was right next to the operating area.

We didn't want that to happen. Thankfully the intravenous injection went in perfectly. After this, as the anaesthetic takes effect, the horse usually wobbles around for a minute or so, before becoming unconscious and sinking to the ground. This has to be carefully managed, to prevent injury to the animal or the handlers. The proximity of the slurry lagoon was still causing us real worry, as we needed to detach the horse from its JCB to allow it to go down safely.

In days gone by, before the routine use of the safe and effective injectable anaesthetics we use today, Mr Sinclair and Pete would perform this procedure using the famous horse chloroform face-mask, which is still in the display cabinet at the practice, next to the 'evil salve'. At that time it was Peter's job, as the junior vet, to get the horse asleep. The canvas mask would be put over the horse's face and nose, and chloroform, a liquid anaesthetic, would be poured onto an absorbent cloth or cotton wool, in the part of the mask nearest the horse's nose. There was little regard paid to the correct dose; it was simply poured in. Once the mask was filled, the horse would be left to wander around a large field, followed by vets and assistants with buckets of water and surgical equipment, waiting for it to fall over. Wherever it fell was the site to perform the operation and it could just as easily be a ditch or an orchard as a flat area of dry, grassy field.

Luckily for us, our drugs had a quicker effect and, after staggering for a few moments, the horse went to ground half way between the digger and the lagoon, so this particular disaster was averted. After this, the surgery was actually the most straightforward part of the morning. We positioned the horse on its side with its uppermost leg pulled forwards to allow Peter to perform the castration. The main concern was that the anaesthetic was sufficiently deep to prevent this leg from twitching or kicking, as the first object it would have met would have been Pete's head. As vets, we have to have quick reactions, but these were not needed today, as the job went perfectly from here. Each testicle was clamped off with special clamps called emasculators, applied to the cord to crush and cut it simultaneously. The blood vessels were ligated and the testicles removed. The only bit to remember during this procedure is to apply the clamps the right way up, otherwise the blood vessels are not clamped and the horse bleeds to death. This very much focuses the mind, but the adage we were taught at vet school, 'nut-to-nut', always helps – it reminds us that the nut on the clamp faces towards the nut on the horse!

As the surgery was completed, everyone involved breathed a collective sigh of relief. It is always preferable for a horse to recover from general anaesthetic as slowly as possible. If it gets up too quickly, it can stumble around in its confused state. Ketamine is used as the anaesthetic and it can cause hallucinations if the pre-op sedative wears off too quickly – and who knows what hallucinations horses experience. Thus, the final part of the job is to supervise the recovery. Everything is not over until the patient is safely standing with slightly spread back legs, nibbling on grass, or in this case, peering optimistically at the mud. It took about twenty minutes for the patient to get up and, as the tension of the morning passed, we chatted amiably to the farmer, caught up on some gossip from the village, and thanked our lucky stars that the animal had avoided the slurry lagoon.

10

My Other Loves

I loved my job in Thirsk. I loved the variety of the work, I loved the North Yorkshire Moors, and I loved being part of the practice. However, I had other loves in my life. My girlfriend, Anne, was working in a rural mixed practice in the Cotswolds. She too had found her ideal job, in a beautiful part of the country, doing the type of work she enjoyed. Perfect, except for the fact that we lived and worked about three and a half hours away from each other, both endlessly busy on call rotas. Most weekends one or other of us would be on call, so whoever was off would make the long Friday-night drive, either north or south, to keep the other one company. Looking back, we coped amazingly well with this situation but, after a couple of years of living separately, it was clear that a solution needed to be found. One of us would need to make a big sacrifice.

The partners in the Cotswold practice didn't want Anne to leave, and the senior partner, Mr Cook, was approaching retirement. We met them one Sunday evening in a lovely little pub in the village of

Winchcombe, where Anne lived. After a brief discussion, they offered me a job. While I was sad to leave Thirsk, a place that had become home, this opportunity was the ideal chance to be with Anne. We could start to make a 'normal' life together after such a long period of being separated by distance and weekend duties. After a brilliant leaving party in the pub in Sutton-under-Whitestonecliffe and an even better meal at Ben's house, we packed the car (it was literally packed, with the cat in her basket wedged up against the roof, surrounded by bags and boxes) and headed south.

The other two loves in my life were the mountains and my mountain bike. Since a vet in rural practice was usually provided with a car and a house, by the age of twenty-seven my most valuable possession in the world was my Scott Expert racing mountain bike. This was securely fastened to the back of the car as we left Thirsk. I had a few months before my job in Winchcombe started, so I had arranged to join a trip biking across the Himalayas. I would be leaving the following weekend. My itinerary involved flying to Lhasa in Tibet, cycling across the Tibetan plateau – 'the roof of the world' – and tracing a path to Kathmandu, the capital of Nepal. In my thirst for the mountains, a visit to the Himalayas had been a long-time dream.

I had been passionate about mountains for as long as I can remember, but my primary love was for climbing them rather than biking through them. I was a very active member of the university climbing club at Cambridge, the CUMC. It was one of the oldest climbing clubs in the country and one with an illustrious heritage. Alumni include the famous British climbers George Mallory, who climbed and was killed on Everest in 1924, and Al Rouse, who was killed on K2 in 1986. As climbers we all knew that danger was a constant presence, but we did everything possible to mitigate the risks. None of us in the CUMC actually thought we would ever be in peril. We felt invincible.

I spent the summer of 1993 climbing in the French and Swiss Alps with friends. The first stop was Chamonix, a Mecca for alpine climbing. I was there with two friends from the university climbing club, Tom and Trish. We had climbed together many times in the wintery mountains of Scotland, around the crags of northern England and the steep sea cliffs of Devon. We wasted no time in getting to grips with the wonderful Frendo spur, which ascends the steep ridge up the Aiguille du Midi, the 3,800-metre spire that dominates the Chamonix valley. We set off from Chamonix and left our tents and supplies at a little lake called Lac Bleu near the base of the steep part of the ridge where the real climbing started. The weather was beautifully clear and the forecast was set fair, so without much concern or discussion, the three of us set off with bivvy bags, ropes, ice axes, ice screws, crampons and everything else we needed to climb this classic. So much for acclimatization – I had only got off the bus an hour previously.

What followed was a series of endless clean and steep pitches of wonderful climbing, on the superb hard, pink granite of the Chamonix valley. It was simply a joy to climb on and we were soon at the top of the rock section and at the bottom of the ice that led up to the knife-sharp ridge connecting the Aiguille du Midi to the Aiguille du Plan. In winter this is the place for serious skiers to negotiate a descent towards the Vallée Blanche, having got to the top via the cable car. It is the highest vertical ascent for a cable car in the world. At this time, this ridge marked safety for the three of us. It is safer to climb ice and snow early in the morning when it has frozen solid. Late afternoon is a dangerous time to be in such places and we had no intention of climbing the next ice stage at five o'clock in the afternoon. Our plan was to bivouac below the icy section and do the hard, steep and exposed bit in the early hours of the morning. We found a great place to set up our bivouac, sheltered from rock fall, and flat so we didn't need to fasten ourselves to the mountain by ropes, which made things slightly more comfortable. It was, however, very cold and without the comfort of a sleeping bag, let alone a tent, we didn't get much sleep.

Morning eventually arrived and, as the sun poked its head up over the Aiguilles Rouges, warmth returned to our limbs. We donned our crampons and climbed, roped together, for the next five hours, using an ice axe in each hand. I had the most experience climbing on ice, so I had to go first. The first of the ice sections was a steep and sharp icy ridge, which led to a final and very exposed snow and ice slope. We moved steadily up the ridge, placing ice screws at intervals. This took us to a steep rock buttress. We traversed underneath this, to the right, taking the opportunity to place safer belays in the rock, as we made our way along the route to the final slopes that led to the summit ridge. This became steeper and steeper. Below us, as I looked down between my legs to check on the progress of Trish and Tom, was an uninterrupted view to the Chamonix valley, three kilometres vertically below. Now would not be the time to mess up.

Eventually, we gained the summit ridge and were met by the strange and slightly disconcerting sight of tourists with cameras who had come up the Aiguille in the cable car. It had been a superb climb, executed to perfection. We celebrated with beers in the café at the summit, before joining the cable car back down. Our feeling of invincibility as climbers increased. We felt we could tackle anything.

Trish returned to the UK soon after this climb but Tom and I did several other classic routes, managing to avoid rock fall on the Grépon and Blaitière, before packing up our kit and heading over the Zermatt – another magnet for climbers – to meet our friend Dave. He had been completing his geology fieldwork in the Alps over the previous month or so, and was desperate to get on with some actual climbing with his mates.

Dave and his geology colleague had been camping in an idyllic alpine pasture with a stream running close by and snow-capped mountains in the background. My basic animal management skills were called upon almost immediately, because their little campsite had been beseiged by brown Swiss cows. They would invade the tents, and after a day of geology, Dave would return to see the 'cow bastards' (his term, not mine) had broken into his tent and eaten all his porridge. Things reached a head when one day they had eaten not only his food, but also his underpants. We soon managed to construct a barrier out of climbing rope, which worked for a time, as the cows thought it was an electric fence.

Tom and Dave had been best friends since school, in Huddersfield, West Yorkshire. I met them both in the CUMC, and got to know Dave during a week of winter ice climbing in a hut in the north of Scotland. He was dry, gruff, honest and said exactly what he thought – a typical Yorkshireman. He was also stocky, handsome and very strong. If he hadn't devoted himself to climbing at university he would have easily filled his time entertaining a very long line of female admirers. Dave and Tom were both very good climbers and much better than I was. The previous summer they had both climbed the Bonatti Pillar on the Aiguille du Dru in Chamonix, one of the hard classics, and it was an epic climb. I hoped I would not be the weakest link in our team of three.

Over the next few days we climbed some of the lower peaks around the Täsch valley near Zermatt. I found I could hold my own in terms of fitness and ability, although the climbs at this part of our trip were not too technically challenging. Our next mission was to tackle the notorious Matterhorn. This was more difficult than anything I had done before. We planned to tackle the hardest ridge – the south-eastern one called the Furggengrat Ridge. This is regarded as harder than the north face of the mountain but a better option in summer, as the faces are usually only climbed in winter when the loose rock is attached firmly by ice. The rock on the Matterhorn is notoriously loose and dangerous and rock fall is the biggest danger to any climber attempting to scale its steep sides.

I was anxious about this route, partly because I was the weakest climber and partly because we were climbing as a three. Steep routes are better climbed in pairs, while groups of three are better suited to less challenging climbs when climbers can 'move together'. This involves being roped together and placing belays every so often. It is much quicker than climbing in a pair, where one person is always fastened, or belayed, to the rock.

We approached the foot of the Matterhorn aiming to bivouac on the lower slopes of the Hörnli Ridge. It took all afternoon to climb to this spot and we reached a suitable place to stop by early evening. By this time the weather forecast had changed and it looked as if we only had one more day of clear weather ahead of us. We had a long discussion about what to do. To embark on the Furggengrat Ridge we would have to start very early, traverse under the eastern face of the mountain, then climb up the very hard ridge. With the weather forecast not stable, we had no flexibility in our plan. We had to be off the mountain by the end of the next day, otherwise we could be stranded if we encountered unforeseen problems. As we looked up at the enormous mountain, it seemed obvious that we should take our chance to climb it, and get off it as quickly as possible. And so we decided to make a quick ascent via the Hörnli Ridge instead. This was technically straightforward and well within our capabilities. We were already on the route and we knew we could climb it easily. The Matterhorn is 4,478 metres high, the sixth highest summit in the Alps, and we were already at about 3,000 metres, near to the Hörnli Hut. While the climbing was continuously steep, with the exception of the top section, we could move together for the vast majority of the route so this seemed the best option. We would be back in the pub before dark. I was secretly quite relieved, although I knew Dave and Tom regretted the missed opportunity to challenge themselves on the hardest route to the summit.

We settled for another uncomfortable night, this time fastened by ropes to the steep rocky sides of the mountain so we didn't roll off in our sleep. Not that there was much sleep, again. The morning sky was grey, rather than the usual alpine bright blue, but it was still and it wasn't snowing. We stashed our sleeping bags and stove under a rock and set off, making quick and steady progress. Because it was cloudy, we only met one other pair of climbers on the whole route. On a sunny day, the route is packed with climbers, which can add another unnecessary risk, so in the absence of this, we felt happy with our decision.

Three-quarters of the way up, we reached a small shed, perched precariously on the north-east ridge at a height of 4,000 metres, called the Solvay Hut. It was named after the Belgian chemist who invented the process for making ammonia, and was built in 1915 to provide shelter for climbers. It had sufficient space to house ten people, if they snuggled up together. It also housed a small radio-telephone in case of emergency. We stopped for a quick drink and rest, and to put on our crampons, before pressing on to the higher and steeper part of the ridge which was covered in ice and hard packed snow. There is a steep section above this area and the rest of the climbing was certainly the hardest part, with snow and ice on the route, but we could easily move together.

Before we knew it, we were standing on the top of the mountain, the wind whistling around our ears and clouds below us. There is a large metal cross on top, as there is on many alpine summits, and we held onto this and whooped with joy. Occasional glimpses of Zermatt and the Hörnli Hut came into view as gaps appeared in the clouds. The summit was so exposed and the sides so steep, that the view was unlike any other I had seen from the top of a mountain. It was like standing at the top of a stepladder. We were never in the habit of lingering on the summit of mountains. Wonderful as these places are, I always felt happier when we reached the safety of lower slopes. We all knew that the most dangerous part of the climb was to come.

We negotiated the steep, icy, upper slopes, using the fixed ropes that had been left in place to make it safer and easier, and moved together with Dave going first. Generally, when moving downwards, the first person is the safest because there are two people on the rope behind to cover in case of a fall. Tom was at the back, because he was still fresh and was the strongest.

Dave moved to the right of the main ridge to lower himself down a small gully off its shoulder. It was exactly the same way we had come up, so we knew it was the correct route. What happened next changed everything forever. Dave manoeuvred himself over a large rock and I was braced in a safe belay stance in case he slipped, with Tom as an extra anchor behind. However, it was the rock that slipped, not Dave, and it rolled downwards with Dave on its underside. It continued sliding and snapped the rope. The rock and Dave fell away, down the eastern face with a terrible thunderous banging as the rock bounced all the way to the bergschrund at the bottom of the face, 3,000 metres below. I pulled on the rope, where Dave should have been, but all that came up was its frayed and severed end. I called Tom. He hadn't seen what had happened because he was just out of sight, over the shoulder of the ridge, but had quickly appeared when he heard the noise. We both shouted Dave's name over and over again, but there was no response. I fired three red emergency flares into the sky and kept my final one for later. No response from anyone.

We had to act quickly. We both knew it would be madness to try and climb down the east face to search for Dave – it was too steep and loose and we knew from the distance that the rock had travelled that he would be a long way down. Our only option was to get to the Solvay Hut as quickly and safely as we could and use the emergency radio-telephone. The hut was about 200 metres below us, directly on the ridge. We were very shaken by now, and we knew the rock was very loose. Our rope was also only about half its original length because it had been severed by the falling rock. We decided to abseil down the route from here. It would be safer but would take longer. With a short rope we estimated it would take eight abseils. After abseiling about three lengths of the rope, we went over an overhang on the ridge. Tom went first and found a safe place to rest and I followed. As I tried to pull the rope through, after getting to the bottom of the section, it got jammed on a piece of protruding rock. This was a disaster and exactly the worst thing that could happen when abseiling. I had to climb back up the rope, using special loops of rope called 'prusik' loops. It was painfully slow and dangerous, but there was no choice.

Eventually, after what seemed like half a day, I managed to dislodge the rope and free it. I returned to the bottom and pulled the rope through. By this time dusk was beginning to set in, but we just managed to reach the hut before it got dark. I called the mountain rescue to let them know what had happened. Very soon afterwards a helicopter was heard flying around the base of the east face. We could just about make out its flashing lights, but we both wept when it flew away after only about ten minutes. We knew they had not found Dave and that they thought any further searching was futile. We sat on the little platform outside the hut, with our legs dangling into space, crying inconsolably. It was desperate. One false move and this had happened. It wasn't even a mistake; we had done everything correctly. It was just horrendous bad luck that the particular rock had moved at the wrong moment. It could have been any one of us, all of us, or none of us.

By now, we all should have been drunk in the bar in Zermatt, as we had planned. Instead, Tom and I spent the next forty-eight hours in this little hut, on the side of the Matterhorn, caught in a blizzard. Life would never be the same again. We had time to think about it all while alone in the hut. In a strange way, it gave us time to come to terms with the accident and the awful loss we had suffered, without distraction or comment from the rest of the world. When I reflect back, while those two days stranded on the mountain were hell, at least we had time to ourselves to gather our thoughts. We felt so sorry for the family and other friends back at home who only heard the news out of the blue over the telephone. They had no time to rationalize what had just happened and mourning must have been much more difficult.

Our attention eventually focused on our own predicament. We had no food or water, no stove to melt snow, no sleeping bags and we were at 4,000 metres in a blizzard with half a rope. Descending would be very dangerous in the soft snow that now lay everywhere. We radioed again, this time to ask to be rescued. Conditions were terrible and at the end of the second day they tried, unsuccessfully, to fly the helicopter to come and get us. It was clearly far too dangerous as visibility was so poor and it was very windy. It was, in reality, only a half-hearted attempt to rescue us but we were in no real danger so we resigned ourselves to a second cold night.

The next day was better and eventually we got a message over the radio to say that rescue was on its way. We were given instructions to put on our harnesses, with screwgate karabiner attached, and to wear helmets and crampons. Our rucksacks should be on and securely fastened. The helicopter finally approached and a man on a winch landed on the little ledge outside our hut. It felt like our hut by now. He deposited a flask of hot orange squash and some ham sandwiches and then disappeared into the sky as the helicopter suddenly lurched upwards. He was only there for a few seconds. We were disappointed at first not to be rescued, and then delighted to have food and hot drink. As we tucked into our feast, the radio burst into life again, saying that they were coming round once more, to try and get us. I went first. The winchman unclipped himself and quickly fastened me onto the winch. The next thing I knew, I was flying around the Matterhorn's north face, almost able to touch it. The winchman was left with Tom and once I was installed in the back seat of this mini helicopter, we returned to get Tom. I can't remember whether we ever did go back to get the man on the end of the winch.

Soon we were back in civilization, in Zermatt, and our predicament became dire again as we realized we had to contact people back home, and first Dave's parents. It was the hardest phone call I have ever had to make.

I haven't climbed serious mountains since then. I have no real intentions of ever doing so again. Six years later I was sitting at Everest base camp with my trusty mountain bike. I was looking up at the highest mountain in the world with a plume of snow travelling horizontally from its top. Once, I would have had a burning urge to be at its summit, but now it looked a very dangerous place to be, and I had absolutely no desire to climb it. The event in 1993 marked a turning point in my life. Dave, one of my closest friends, with whom I had shared some wonderful times, was dead and life could no longer be the same. I was about to start my clinical studies at vet school, exactly half way through my university course. So, with memories of Dave constantly present, the focus of my life shifted away from the mountains, and towards veterinary medicine in earnest.

11

A Year in the Cotswolds

My biking trip through the Himalayas was superb. I had worked very hard for those first three years in practice and, while I had loved it, I was very much in need of a break. A month amongst the biggest mountains on earth was the perfect antidote and I relished every moment. We covered up to 60 miles on our mountain bikes every day, climbing up and over passes of over 5,000 metres in altitude, in maybe the most awe-inspiring surroundings that the world has to offer. It was mind-expanding and energizing, and I was hungry for more veterinary work when I returned.

Anne came to collect me from the airport. Soon, our conversation turned to what was next. I had three months before I was due to start work at Anne's practice in the Cotswolds, so my plan was to find a locum job for the intervening period. Locum work is sometimes regarded as a 'rite of passage' for young vets and many would use it as an opportunity to travel to Australia or New Zealand. I had no desire to work so far afield – Anne and I had been apart for too long already.

Anne had been in charge of contacting locum agencies on my behalf while I had been away. She had found a possible position with a vet called Nick, who ran a small practice in the Forest of Dean. He sounded very keen to meet me, so the very next day, I got back on my bike and cycled from Winchcombe to meet him at his practice. Since I was between jobs I had no car (my old red Metro had been put into retirement some years previously), so my trusty but rather dusty mountain bike was the only means of transport. It was a long way, but I was full of energy, having been at altitude for the last four weeks and used to cycling 60 miles a day over very rough terrain. I was very fit and my blood cells were boosted. However, I also had a terrible bowel infection, acquired while recovering from our epic bike ride, in Kathmandu. As a result, my ride to the Forest of Dean was punctuated by regular stops at any public conveniences I could find. Despite this rather unconventional approach to an interview, Nick offered me a temporary job to help with cover over the summer holidays.

I didn't know much about the Forest of Dean. It proved to be a lovely but rather peculiar place. Its idiosyncrasies took me somewhat by surprise. The forest is situated on a small coal seam and is littered with small, disused coal mines dating back to the nineteenth and early twentieth centuries. Coming from a mining town in West Yorkshire, I thought I knew about coal mining, but what happened here was a world away from the large-scale operations on the huge coalfaces of south Wales and the north of England. Here, the rules were different, and individuals who qualified were granted leases to mine in certain areas, under a system called 'free mining'. The enormous advances in technology that occurred during the industrial revolution seemed to have bypassed the forest, and in the mid-nineteenth century this small area alone had over three hundred small mines. Very few are still producing coal, but many disused mine shafts remain, dotted around the forest, each one recognizable by a small opening heading horizontally into the hillside. They look just like the ones that are full of ghosts in *Scooby Doo*.

In the towns and villages of the forest, there was still the atmosphere of a pre-industrial era. I was once standing at the cash machine outside the bank, when three sheep walked up and stood behind me in the queue! It made Thurso look like a bustling metropolis, and Thirsk too.

It was a great place to spend a summer and an insight into a different type of veterinary work. The practice solely dealt with small animals, and was very businesslike. I learnt a lot about how to run the financial side of a practice, since for much of the time I was in sole charge while the boss was on holiday. The best bit of the job, however, was that I had a full two-hour break at lunchtime. I was used to about twenty minutes for lunch on a good day back in Thirsk, so this was a real luxury. I usually took my bike and used the time to go mountain biking around the forest. I also only worked a four-day week, so I had plenty of time to explore this new part of the country.

One day I was returning from my usual lunchtime circuit in the forest when I came across an injured cat by the side of the road. I had nothing other than a bike pump and a puncture repair kit with me, which I did not think would be very helpful to this poor cat. It was obviously in a very bad way. It had severe head injuries and bleeding, bulging eyes. The only thing I could do was to scoop it up and ride back to the practice as quickly as possible. It was about a ten-minute ride, mainly downhill, so I sped off as fast as I could. The cat didn't like being held and despite its injuries made vigorous attempts to escape. It was also hard to hold a cat and ride fast downhill, so I stopped my bike and 'scruffed' the cat with one hand. This is a way of controlling a cat safely, by firmly grasping the fold of skin on the back of its neck. While it looks unkind, it is completely painless and is the way a mother cat holds onto her baby kittens. It also keeps a cat with flailing claws and teeth a safe distance away from the handler.

As I whizzed downhill at high speed to get back to the oxygen machine, x-rays, intravenous fluids and other medication, I couldn't help but notice the strange looks I was getting from the cars that were overtaking me. Some drivers were even gesticulating at me with their fists. I think they must have thought that I was taking my cat for some kind of weird cycling experience, completely against its will. Other drivers, however, appeared utterly oblivious to my cat-cycling antics. Like I said, the forest is a peculiar place. The cat made a good recovery, but had used up one of its nine lives.

———

In the course of our veterinary lives, Anne and I had both been consulted on many occasions about dogs that chewed the house, puppies that wouldn't house train or who destroyed shoes, clothes or furniture. On close questioning, it often emerged that these animals were left on their own for long periods of time. It was always surprising to us that some owners seemed to expect a five-month-old puppy to hang on all day without a wee, or were outraged when it sought some comfort from its absent owner's lovely smelly footwear. Consequently, even though we both longed for a dog, we had decided this would be entirely inappropriate while we were still commuting between Thirsk and Winchcombe every weekend, and working long hours on duty. However, now that we were finally in one place, the time seemed, at last, to be right, and Paddy the border terrier came into our life. Anne went up to collect him from Ripon on her half day. He was a tiny, ten-week-old ball of fluff, just like a teddy bear. We introduced him to our little black cat, Billy, who promptly hit him on the nose with her paw. Our cottage was also tiny, with no place for either cat or dog to escape from one another, so they had to learn to get on. Paddy forgave the cat her initial punch on the nose and tried to make friends, but the cat never really returned the sentiment, although a tolerance of sorts eventually developed. In one early encounter, Paddy came rushing in and enthusiastically chased the cat upstairs. She made a beeline for the bathroom window and flung herself out. Clearly she was desperate to escape. We spent hours searching for her, convinced she must be mortally wounded, but she sauntered in at three in the morning as if nothing had happened. It took her a while to realize that, if she didn't run, Paddy wouldn't chase her. If she stood her ground, he just wagged his tail and eventually wandered off, slightly confused.

Paddy was a great little dog and he had a brilliant place to grow up. We lived in a beautiful street in Winchcombe called Vineyard Street. It is probably one of the most picturesque streets in Britain, leading up to Sudeley Castle, the burial place of Catherine Parr, the sixth wife of Henry VIII, and home to Edward VI and Thomas Seymour. History oozed from every part of its grounds, where we took little Paddy for his first walks. He grew up to be a handsome and proud terrier, but at this time he was full of fun and played constantly. On one of his early walks he misjudged a cattle grid over which he thought he could jump, and landed, splat, in the middle. He hobbled home, badly lame. The only thing to do was to take an x-ray. This was the first time we had the responsibility of tending to our own pet and it felt slightly strange. We identified a hairline crack in his radius and, as was normal procedure, bandaged it up in a sturdy bandage. We knew that a tiny fracture in a youngster would heal in just a few weeks, with this kind of simple and non-invasive treatment. Unfortunately, poor Paddy looked miserably sad with his enormous bandage and he stubbornly refused to walk or even move with his bandaged leg. We could not bear to see him looking so gloomy, and removed the bandage after only forty-eight hours. We had utterly disregarded our very own veterinary advice, purely because of his sad face. His leg, however, did heal quite quickly and he was soon back in action around the lovely footpaths of the Cotswolds.

My locum job in the Forest of Dean ended after a couple of months, and I started my new position, working alongside Anne. It was great to be back in mixed practice, where I had chance to get out onto farms and to see horses again. However, I had to become familiar with the area and get to know the farmers and horse owners from scratch. I had developed many friendships in Thirsk, but down here I had to start again, find new friends in the farming community and establish my reputation.

This was easier than previously because I had quite a bit of experience, but my first few weeks and months were not completely free of problems. On one occasion I had been called to see a lame horse. Little Paddy was with me and jumped out of the car as soon as I arrived on the yard. I asked if it was okay for him to potter around while I attended to the horse. It provided the little pup with a fun-packed morning if he could snuffle around after bits of horse hoof trimmings. The lady suggested it would be better if he stayed in the car, because she had a new collection of small and very expensive rare breed ducklings. Once older, these birds would lay special blue eggs and they had been a present from her husband.

I left him in the car, watching me through the window, as I dealt with the horse. I pared its foot with my hoof knives and released the pocket of pus that was causing its pain. 'Great,' I thought, as it is immensely satisfying when you find that place that has been causing so much discomfort. Dark grey, fetid-smelling liquid shot out of the hole that I had just excavated in the sole of the horse's foot. When I went back to get some bandages from my car boot, Paddy jumped out again. I ushered him back into the car, but the lady had obviously realized that he was far too cute to be a threat to the new ducklings, and waved her hand as if to say, 'Don't worry, it will be fine.'

I turned my attention back to the foot, and carefully applied the dressing, which looked very neat and tidy by the time I had finished. The horse was already much more comfortable and, as its owner walked it back to the stable, it did not even seem to be lame. Job done, I looked around to find the dog.

'Paddy! ... Paddy! ... *PADDY!*'

After a few minutes, which felt more like an hour, the little dog reappeared with his head held high and his tail up. He looked very pleased with himself. He also had a beautiful and expensive duckling sticking out of his mouth. There was much quacking and commotion. I extracted the dishevelled bird, quickly examined it, deposited it back on the pond, bundled Paddy into the car and made a very quick getaway. I did not stop to see whether it floated back to its mum or sank to the bottom of the pond.

This was Paddy's first misdemeanour, but not his last. We had not learnt our lesson. A few months later, dog in car, I set off to see a bull that had died suddenly. I had been summoned to perform a post mortem examination to establish the cause of its demise. Having ruled out anthrax (I had at least, learnt my lesson in this regard), I embarked upon the post mortem. Paddy was, again, safely shut in, watching my every move through the car window. I cut through skin and muscle and was soon scooping out the abdominal contents like some sort of medieval soothsayer. I found nothing abnormal, so turned my attention to the chest cavity. This is the hardest part because of the thick ribs, and I really needed the equipment of a butcher rather than the precision instruments of a surgeon. Nevertheless, I managed to cut a window in the ribs of sufficient size to remove the heart and lungs, which I examined carefully. It was clear that the animal had died of acute pneumonia. I explained this to the worried farmer as I gathered my stethoscope and thermometer from the car. It was likely the dead bull was the tip of the pneumonic iceberg, so I needed to examine the other beasts in the group, and treat them promptly to avoid further losses. As I set about the task, I was sure I had closed the boot of the car fully.

Forty-five minutes later, I returned to collect a bucket and brush to clean my wellies. No dog. He had clearly sneaked out of the car when I went to see the other animals. He was nowhere to be seen but I was not especially worried, so I continued to scrub my boots and wash my hands under the tap. He would show up. And indeed, after a few calls, Paddy obediently appeared. But he appeared right out of the middle of the bull carcass and he was completely covered in blood. Very red blood – all over his head, body and feet, and dribbling from the corners of his mouth. It was just as if he had been dipped in bright red paint. I could not believe my eyes. I was astonished and cross, but I didn't need to raise my voice: he knew he had been bad and pretty much took himself off, to stand under the hosepipe for a very thorough cleaning.

Paddy's adventures continued and he became a popular character in the village. It was a short walk from our house in Vineyard Street to the branch surgery, where I was based. Next door to the surgery was a pub called the Plaisterers Arms, then the doctor's surgery and then the bank. In those child-free days, we would often call in at the Plaisterers Arms for a pint, a chat with Ken, the Irish landlord, or a game of darts after finishing evening surgery. In fact, when we walked up the road with Paddy, he would stop at the door of the practice, but if we weren't going in there, he would automatically take himself to the pub. Late one evening, a few days after the incident with the bull, Ken had drunk one too many halves of Guinness. He was firm in his opinion that a bit of stout did a dog a world of good. Anne and I returned from the dartboard to see our dog sitting contentedly, licking his furry, foam-covered whiskers, next to an empty drip tray. The drip tray had been catching the overflow from glasses of Guinness all night. It was the second time that week that he had the air of achievement about his canine person. Knowing about pharmacology and also about drinking, it was clear that half a pint of stout to a six-kilogram dog was the equivalent of a fifteen-year-old boy drinking about ten pints. It was too late to do much about it, though, and so all we could do was take him home. The poor dog meandered along on his lead, urinating about every ten paces and wobbling while he did so. Eventually we made it the short distance back. If Paddy could have spoken, he would have assured us both that he really, really loved us.

The next morning Paddy didn't move from his bed. I bundled him up and carried him to the practice. He headed straight to the dog bed under the desk in reception, and hid his head under the blanket. Clearly the poor dog had a hangover and I felt terrible. I offered him painkillers and oral rehydration drinks and by lunchtime he was feeling much better, though he wasn't in quite such a rush to go back into the Plaisterers Arms the next night. I feel sure that he was not the first 'Paddy' to be on the wrong end of the landlord's generous hospitality!

———

Work was great, and it was brilliant being able to spend time with Anne after too many years in separate parts of the country. This is a common problem for veterinary couples. The veterinary degree course is long, and veterinary students spend many hours working intensively alongside one another, so it is not unusual for vets to end up in relationships with other vets. In some ways this is helpful. People who are not familiar with the nature of the job and its utter commitment, in terms of hours on call and weekends tied up and busy, might find it very difficult to live with a vet. Add to that smelly and muddy cars, blood-stained shirts, chronic fatigue and a persistent low-grade bad temper when woken up too many times during the night, and vets could be considered not to make the best of partners.

In other ways, two vets in a relationship can pose a big problem. Vets in mixed practice have to live close to their surgery, so they can be there to treat an emergency as quickly as possible. It is, therefore, not really possible to commute, and finding two jobs close enough together is difficult. Often, big compromises or sacrifices are needed from one or both sides of the relationship. We were extremely lucky to have managed to get jobs in the same practice. At last, the miserable Sunday-night journey up or down the M42 was a thing of the past, and we could live together, which was wonderful.

We worked together very well, with hardly any squabbles, either professionally or personally. Our professional attitudes were very similar. We both had a pragmatic and straightforward approach to work and to clinical cases. Jobs needed doing and animals needed to be treated, and the only way was to get on and do it. There was no room for avoiding hard work or ducking the challenging jobs. After all, we both saw clearly that this was how to learn and progress.

One night, Anne was called to a calving at a large beef herd just outside Broadway. Calls to this particular farm were usually tough, and often necessitated two vets. Since the beeper had woken me up as well, it seemed silly to drag the vet on second call out of his bed, and I offered to go along in case a caesarean was needed.

Sure enough, this calf was not budging and we performed the operation together, under the light of head torches, in the middle of a freezing cow shed in the middle of the night. It was the first time we had operated on a cow together, but it did not feel like a romantic moment.

The Cotswolds was a beautiful place to be, the type of work was very similar to what I was used to, and I felt at home. There were some differences, though. I had many more horses to see, which really improved my equine expertise. Clients were much the same.

People often talk about the differences between 'northerners' and 'southerners' and how one group is friendlier than the other. In my experience this is complete nonsense. There are friendly, happy, kind and sociable people everywhere, just as there are miserable, grumpy and intolerant people. Being in one part of the country rather than another does not mean an exclusivity of any of these features or characteristics. That said, in this part of the country, there were many large houses owned by wealthy people who spent the working week in London, and this would leave some of the villages somewhat empty and lacking in atmosphere during the week. By contrast in Thirsk, pretty much everyone lived and worked in the area so the villages had a much more cohesive atmosphere.

One other difference I noticed was the number of elderly lady clients who lived alone in enormous houses. There were often photographs suggesting a glamorous past, usually involving racehorses, as we were close to Cheltenham, and sometimes there was a vintage Bentley parked – rarely used – in the garage. One particular such client had a small dachshund called Sebastian, which had a bad back. Whenever the little dog needed attention (which was often), we would be asked to do a house visit. 'Mornings are better for me,' was her usual comment when visits were being arranged. As a newcomer to these parts, I did not immediately grasp the significance of this request. I assumed she had an important voluntary job at the local church or played bridge in the afternoons. As often as possible, we complied with her requests, but one day my morning visit was delayed. I had been busy with a tuberculosis test on twelve cows. I was expecting the test to take about half an hour, but when I arrived I was dismayed to see all twelve cattle happily grazing in the field next to the farm. It was a large field surrounded by a hedge. This hedge had holes in and there was only a very flimsy fence. To cut a very long story short, the cows did not want to be captured. We chased them around the field, the adjacent fields, the farmyard, the slurry lagoon, the silage clamp and a nearby wood. Three hours later it became clear that this was an impossible job and with red faces and frayed tempers, the farmer and I admitted defeat. We would have to rearrange the test for another occasion, when the cattle had already been caught.

It was well into the afternoon by this point, and I was very late for my visit to Sebastian the dachshund. I made my way up the long drive and knocked on the supersized door, apologizing profusely for my lateness as the housekeeper showed me into the sitting room. Mrs B was sitting comfortably in a large chair with a tray on a small table next to her. On this was a half-pint-sized tumbler, a saucer with sliced lemons, two bottles of tonic and a bottle of gin. Half of the gin was already missing.

'Ah, thank you for coming, are you the new vet?' she slurred. We had met several times before, so either our first meetings had left no impression at all, or the old lady could not remember. Before I could offer more apologies for arriving on the wrong side of midday, Mrs B went on to explain the problem with the dog. 'It's his todger,' she blurted out rather bluntly.

'Oh, I see. I'll have a look.'

Being a dachshund, Sebastian had very short legs and the hind ones were weak, because of his back problems. This meant that the poor dog's penis did, on occasions, rub along the ground or worse, get caught on the side of his wicker basket as he pulled himself in or out. It was very sore, and made worse by his constant licking. Dogs like to lick this part of their anatomy at the best of times, but any wound or soreness gives extra impetus to this canine pastime. He needed a combination of antibiotics and cream to be applied twice daily. I carefully explained the treatment to both the old lady and the housekeeper, as I was not confident that my instructions would be clearly remembered by the next morning.

Later that evening, when I recounted my story to Anne, there was much mirth. Anne had been working at the practice for two years already, and she knew full well the significance of the phrase 'mornings are better for me'. She also knew that it was unwise to arrange any visits after a TB test to Mr Wilson's.

We always discussed our day's work when we sat down to eat in the evening. It was great to be able to do this in person, rather than over the telephone, as we had been used to for the last few years. In fact, twenty years later, it is something we still do. It probably sounds tedious, but it is a really good way to get a different perspective on a case, air one's frustrations or get new ideas on a treatment. One evening, Anne related the tale of her day spent dehorning and castrating a bunch of about forty wild calves at an exposed farm near the top of a hill. The elderly farmer always drafted in the help of his equally elderly neighbour for this annual task, which often took two days. I had been to the farm once, to do the same job on a day when it rained constantly. Mud was everywhere and the pen holding the cattle was in the middle of the mud. The cattle crush was also surrounded by mud and there was no shelter anywhere. It was always a tough job and the cattle were not used to being handled.

The animals, as usual, varied in size from fairly small to way too big. To begin with they were all milling about in the mud, but the plan was to herd them, in batches, into a stable, from where they could be funnelled down a race into the crush. It was the job of the elderly neighbour to push them down the race. He did this, not particularly effectively, with a lot of shouting, swearing and waving of his stick. The biggest beast was not keen to be caught. It was eventually corralled into the stable towards the end of the day, and proceeded to cause havoc, hurling itself around and generally making life difficult. The shouting, swearing and flapping of arms suddenly ended with an expletive, as the beast kicked out and caught the old man. Those waiting at the crush to deal with the last of the animals weren't particularly sympathetic, as everyone just wanted to get the job finished and get home. Once it was all done, Anne went back to her car to sort out her kit and the injured neighbour took himself off to examine his wounds.

'Can you just have a look at this?' came a wavering voice from behind a tractor. Anne followed the voice, to find the old man, white as a sheet, trousers round his ankles, inspecting an enormous purple haematoma about an inch wide, running all the way from his groin to his knee. The unruly young bullock had kicked out and caught the end of the stick, ramming it down the inside of the poor man's leg, which had caused the massive blistering bruise. Anne peered at the wound with a clinician's eye, but just as she began to suggest a cream of some sort, she realized the ludicrous nature of the scene. There she was, behind a tractor, with an old man with his trousers down, examining his inner thigh … she briskly extricated herself from the situation, and decided this might be someone else's job next year.

The story of a young, attractive female vet, examining the upper, inner thigh of a farmer, behind a tractor, with his trousers round his ankles, could have become a legend of Arthurian proportions, and it would make a great story if this was the reason for us moving away from the Cotswolds and back up to Yorkshire. But it isn't. Fate had intervened again and, back up in Thirsk, Jim was looking for someone to buy his share of the partnership at Skeldale. This would give me the opportunity to become junior partner at the practice. Life was about to change direction again.

12

Back in Thirsk

The opportunity to buy into a veterinary practice is an exciting prospect, but also a daunting one. It brings with it a huge financial burden and a lifetime of commitment. As I discussed the situation with Pete, he likened it to a marriage. He was right in many ways.

Suddenly, Anne and I had a lot of decisions to make. We had expected to be fairly settled for the next few years, living in Winchcombe, but now there was the chance of a long-term investment in our future which, hopefully, once the enormous business loan had been repaid, would put us in a robust position for the rest of our lives. Once we started to discuss this, we thought it only fair to bring it to the attention of the partners of the practice where we were working. To their enormous credit, they quickly made us the offer of a partnership in their practice. This added another twist to our situation, especially as Anne loved her job immensely, and could see her own future there, as a partner.

After many evenings of debate and countless nights of broken sleep, we eventually made the decision to make the move back up north. We needed a house, and I set about the arrangement of a business loan, to pay for the partnership. The constraints of our rota meant that we were only off together one weekend in five, so house hunting was tricky. I made the journey alone on one occasion and, after looking at a couple of properties and taking lots of photographs, we made an offer on an end-of-terrace house. Anne hadn't even seen it at this point, apart from via my not very professional photos. It was a bold move and one that seemed rash when we both did eventually manage to visit Thirsk to look at the house together.

We had been at a wedding in Cambridge on a Friday evening in early December, and made the trip from Cambridge to Yorkshire on a gloomy Saturday morning. It was a journey I had made many times, but this was the first time I had done it with a view to inspecting our future house, and indeed, our actual future. Thirsk could not have looked a more terrible place to move to, on this particular day. It looked a world away from the beautiful Cotwolds. Everything was dark grey and mist hung heavily in the air. Thirsk is on the edge of the North York moors but also at the end of the wide, flat Vale of York, so fog and damp lingers here on a bad day in winter. This was such a day and although I loved the area, even I had to admit that it looked rubbish. Anne managed to put a brave face on it, and we pressed on with the purchase of the house. Three months later I was back in Thirsk for good, back in my old patch. Last time I was here, my most valuable possession was a mountain bike. Now, I owned a house and part of a practice, and I owed a whole load of money in all directions. It was the start of a new millennium and everything was exciting, if daunting.

Anne stayed on for a few months in Winchcombe, so that the practice wasn't left suddenly short of two vets. I felt responsible for 'stealing' their dynamic assistant, Anne. It was only fair she should stay on for a while. I embarked enthusiastically on all sorts of DIY projects in the new house. This was dangerous without direct supervision from Anne, as I am not known for my fantastic DIY skills. Painting was OK and I actually managed to get most of the house decorated before Anne moved up.

The grouting of the hall tiles was altogether different, though.

One weekend we decided we would lay quarry tiles in our new entrance hall. It was more of a job than we expected, as our tile cutter wasn't up to cutting the solid tiles, and we had to hire a power tool. Anne returned to the Cotswolds on Sunday night, suggesting we leave the grouting until she was up next, three weeks later. She didn't seem entirely convinced by my assurance that I knew what I was doing, but I was determined to get the grouting completed before her return. How hard could it be? I smeared the concrete-like mixture into all the gaps between the tiles on Friday evening, after I had finished work, then headed back down to see Anne for the weekend. When I arrived, I enthusiastically explained my progress with the tiles, how I had left it all to dry and my plans to wipe off the excess on my return to Thirsk on Sunday. Anne's ashen face made me think this would not be so straightforward. Sure enough, the grouting had set like rock and the mixture, which I was planning to wipe off with a cloth, was cemented on, rock hard and immovable. It took the next two weeks and many rolls of wire wool to solve the problem. With good reason, I have never been asked to do a serious DIY job again.

Before long, Anne was up in Yorkshire for good. The old problem of finding the right sort of work close by reared its head again, but she managed to secure two part-time jobs in nearby practices, and we settled down to our new life. We were also engaged to be married, and Anne's parents had enthusiastically been looking at venues for a wedding in late springtime of the same year. To the disappointment of Anne's father, we quickly realized that buying a house, moving to the opposite end of the country, buying into a business and getting married all in the space of a few months was not going to be possible. However, we found a date in October that was perfect. It was a lovely autumnal day in rural Hampshire (Anne's childhood home) – damp and misty but so calm and serene. I went for a mountain bike ride very early in the morning with my mates Ben L and Ben C, and my best man, Mike (the funniest man I know – he did me justice with his speech that day). The bike ride did a lot to steady the nerves. The day went so quickly and with jaws sore from smiling and talking so much, we all enjoyed cigars later that evening. If being a partner was like being married, I thought, it was going to be a doddle.

I hadn't really appreciated that being a partner in a practice also meant running the business. We had received expert training at vet school in how to be a veterinary surgeon – examination, diagnosis and treatment of all manner of diseases and injuries and all types of animal. Nobody had given us any training on how to make a business work. I quickly realized that I had very much to learn. Until this point in my career, my only priority had been the treatment of my patients. Now I had to make sure that we could pay our staff and our massive monthly bills for drugs, rates and insurance as well as new equipment and repairs to old equipment. The repairs and maintenance to our dental machine would regularly cost several hundred pounds. Since, at this time, we charged about £50 for a dental, after taking off other costs, we needed to do about ten dentals a month just to pay for the machine's regular maintenance. Running the x-ray processor was even worse. On top of this, Anne and I had a mortgage and I had a hefty business loan. Financial pressures were suddenly huge, and it made work, for the first time, very stressful. I devised a system of measuring the cost of something in terms of 'how many anal glands' it equated to. Anal glands are a major design fault in the dog and they pose a daily, smelly challenge to vets. The glands are marble-sized structures on either side of the anus, which fill up with foul-smelling pasty liquid. Their purpose is to scent mark, but sometimes they don't empty properly and the full anal glands can cause discomfort or sometimes great pain. Occasionally the contents leak out onto the sofa or onto the owner's trousers, which causes just as much distress to the owner. I cannot recall a working day that hasn't involved emptying some anal glands at some point. It is a simple but unpleasant job and we charged about £5 for such a procedure. Therefore a new autoclave machine (used for sterilizing surgical kit) that cost £8,000 would be equivalent to emptying about 1,600 anal glands. It was a useful way to quantify costs, but I dared not calculate the anal gland equivalent of my business loan!

Contrary to popular opinion, most veterinary surgeons do not earn huge salaries. The majority of vets in private practice work, primarily, for the benefit of their animal patients. The financial motivation is not, generally, a primary factor. We would rather treat an animal and make it better than earn an enormous salary. Our margins are pretty narrow, especially on drug sales, and our typical mark-up on most dispensed drugs is twenty per cent. I quickly realized that this did not give much room for wastage. If we buy a bottle of shampoo for £10, and sell it for £12, we make £2 profit. If one bottle gets wasted, or is used and not charged for, we lose £10. Therefore, to break even on the shampoo, we need to sell another five bottles. The pair of artery forceps that falls into the straw and gets lost during a caesarean on a sheep, costs more than the price we charge for doing the operation in the first place, and the bottle of antibiotics that falls off the cattle crush and smashes on the floor costs £158. All these figures I can now pluck out of my head, but as an assistant I had no idea how much things cost or how much impact this wastage had on the practice finances. During my first few years as a partner I lost many hours of sleep, worrying about what I had bought into, my enormous debt and the stability of our future. I do not think I was the only vet in the country with such nocturnal anxiety – it is well known that the veterinary profession has one of the highest suicide rates of any of the professions. This may be more to do with ease of access to drugs used for euthanasia, but must also be, in part, due to these financial worries.

The other major problem facing veterinary practices was, and is, that of the outstanding debt, owed by clients who have not paid for the veterinary attention they have received. Since our first and foremost priority is always the health and welfare of animals, we are often stung by individuals who have sick animals but no intention of paying. It is a huge burden, particularly for large animal and mixed practices, and it is miraculous that many still exist as businesses at all. We still have several farms that owe us many thousands of pounds. One has not paid us anything for over four years. I went there in 2006 to replace a prolapsed uterus in a cow. It was after midnight and the middle of winter. I was completely asleep when my beeper went off, and it almost didn't wake me. A prolapsed uterus is very urgent and needs immediate attention. It was pretty serious, and I attended to the cow, replaced the uterus and gave all the necessary medication. To this day, the practice has not been paid for my work, ten years later.

It was not all doom and gloom, though. In fact the financial pressure was really the only negative thing about being a partner, and I was slowly developing ways of handling these new pressures, mainly in the form of gin and tonic. Life was good and married life was great. We were enjoying the fun of bringing up our young border terrier, Paddy, who was now approaching adolescence. Free weekends usually involved long dog walks on the moors or in the Dales, and Paddy was a great companion as Anne and I explored all the paths and byways of this lovely area. Two or three times his youthful exuberance got the better of him as he raced off into the woods, chasing deer, then got completely lost. On all these occasions, we spent hours searching with torches as it got dark. Eventually he would turn up, exhausted and muddy after his adventures, at a house nearby. We learnt that the best strategy was for one of us to go home to sit by the phone, while the other searched.

Our house was in a village on the outskirts of Thirsk, which Paddy was beginning to consider his own. He was a lovely, friendly dog, but he was starting to see younger, male dogs as challengers to his self-appointed status as the top dog in the village. One Monday afternoon, his attempts at village dominance became too much. As I stood chatting to the owner of a younger male dog, Paddy growled, snarled and then rushed at the pup, intent on attacking him.

'This will not do,' I thought. I could not let him attack the other dogs in the neighbourhood; it was a terrible example to set to the local dog-owning community. So, we marched him straight round to the practice to remove his testicles. Anne and I both knew that castrating him was the best solution for a young male dog who was beginning to show his dominance. Wasting no time, we dosed him with his pre-med (the pre-anaesthetic sedation given to patients prior to the actual anaesthetic). Little Paddy seemed to be more sensitive to the sedative than most dogs. He wobbled and swayed all over the prep room, seeming not to realize that his legs were going in different directions, before I gave him his anaesthetic.

As a vet, operating on your own animal is a tricky dilemma. On the one hand, you don't really want to trust anyone else with your beloved pet, or give them that burden of responsibility. On the other, you are very much less detached than normal, and this can often lead to mistakes or complications that would never otherwise happen. Some vets (including my wife) absolutely refuse to operate on, or treat their own dogs. One colleague was castrating his parents' dog, also a border terrier, when the most freakish accident happened. An unligated blood vessel recoiled back into his abdomen, squirting blood internally like an out of control hosepipe. It took three of us, and major abdominal surgery to rectify the situation.

So, I embarked on the process with just a small amount of trepidation. It was the first time I had needed to operate on my own animal. Having given him the anaesthetic induction agent by injection, I inserted a breathing tube to provide oxygen and the gas that would keep him asleep while I operated. All went as normal. It happened that on that particular day, a new head nurse had started, and she was keen to impress. She had taken apart and thoroughly cleaned our two anaesthetic circuits and left them to dry during the afternoon. When I blustered in with my dog, needing a seemingly emergency castration, she had quickly reassembled the circuits, ready for the procedure. I connected Paddy to the anaesthetic machine, but no oxygen flowed down his tube and after a few moments the circuit shot off the machine like a cork shooting out of a bottle of fizzy wine. I had never seen this happen before and immediately replaced the circuit with the other one. The same thing happened, and the circuit fired off the machine yet again. Anne, who was monitoring Paddy's anaesthetic, started to verge on panic, and I started shouting. This was very irregular and not at all what should be happening to any dog, let alone my own beloved pet. The third circuit we tried worked fine and the rest of the operation proceeded without complication. As the little dog slowly recovered from the procedure, we investigated the cause of problem. It became clear that one short length of tube in each circuit had been connected the wrong way round, so the flow of oxygen through the circuit was not possible. Our new nurse was mortified and very apologetic. No harm was done, but needless to say, this simple mistake did not happen again!

Paddy made an uneventful recovery, quite oblivious to the anxiety that had ensued during the operation. He rested quietly that evening, feeling very sorry for himself and probably presuming it was yet another hangover. The positive effect on his behaviour with other male dogs was instant, and never again did he even so much as bare his teeth to another dog. That is until we introduced him, only a couple of years ago, to our tiny new puppy, Emmy. By that time he had reached a great old age, and was not even slightly impressed at this young intruder trying to climb into bed with him.

While my first year as a business owner had been challenging, and an exciting learning process, I eventually began to realize that coming back to Thirsk had been a sensible move. I could see that my debts would eventually be paid off, and, despite the money owed to us by too many farmers, the future was rosy. I was becoming an accomplished veterinary surgeon, I was learning the ropes of practice management and I generally felt optimistic about the future of the practice, and for Anne and me.

However, on 19 February 2001, the turn of events made it seem likely that the face of farming in Britain, and of rural mixed practice, might change forever.

13

Foot-and-Mouth Disease – a Return to the Dark Ages

On Friday 19 February 2001, a suspected case of foot-and-mouth disease was reported at an abattoir in Essex. A veterinary inspector had identified suspicious lesions in a pig as it stood, drooling, in the lairage. These were the days before the rapid dissemination of information via email and the internet, and we received the news by fax from MAFF. MAFF stood for the Ministry of Agriculture, Fisheries and Food. It was the government department responsible for overseeing the health of the nation's livestock, both in terms of animal welfare and disease control.

The news was clearly alarming. Foot-and-mouth disease is extremely infectious, causing severely debilitating illness in many animals, very quickly. It had not been seen in the UK since 1968. It seemed like an old-fashioned disease, and was not something that the majority of practising vets had ever seen, although we had all learnt about it in detail at vet school. Jim Wight had been involved in the previous outbreak, so was immediately sent off to Staffordshire to help with the control measures, even though he, like most of his cohort of veterinary surgeons, had recently hung up his stethoscope. Most of our knowledge was, therefore, based around black and white photos of desperate-looking cattle attended by vets with serious faces and long, black, plastic coats that reached to their feet.

Pete, Tim and I knew that this was a potentially serious situation for the country, and for the farming and veterinary industries, but Essex was a long way away and we were not really aware of the full implications of the outbreak. However, Stewart, a perpetually cheerful Scottish vet who was working with us at the time, had previously been employed by MAFF as a veterinary investigations officer. As part of his training, he had learnt much about foot-and-mouth, and he fully understood how grave things were. He was going on holiday skiing for a week the very next day, and his parting comment as he bade us farewell was, 'Oh, lads, this is gonna be really bad. Things will not be the same when I get back from Austria.'

How right he was. By the following day, the disease had been confirmed officially, and the proverbial had hit the fan. MAFF imposed a movement ban in the area around the infected premises, making it illegal to move any animals, even to a nearby field. By Tuesday of the following week, this movement ban had become nationwide. It became clear that the disease had become widely disseminated even before the first case had been identified, as cases started to appear as far afield as Devon and Cumbria. There was a rapid and dramatic escalation of cases, footpaths were closed and the countryside, and in fact the whole country, ground to a very dazed and stunned halt. Nobody really knew what was happening or what was going to happen. Our farm work immediately stopped. One farmer phoned up to ask me to go and do a routine fertility on his dairy herd and was somewhat bemused when I explained that we would have to postpone any non-urgent visits, as we didn't want to risk any possible disease spread by undertaking any visits to farms that were not emergencies.

This was a period, around Thirsk at least, that was akin to the 'phoney war' of 1939, after Britain had declared war on Germany but nothing really happened. We simply watched the news and the fax machine for unfolding events. So far, at least, our area and our clients were largely unaffected.

That was, of course, apart from the movement restrictions and their consequences. Obviously it is not possible to completely stop the movement of livestock around the country. Sheep needed to be moved back to farms from the hills and far-flung fields so they could be lambed under supervision, pigs and fattening cattle needed to be moved to slaughter as they achieved their finishing weight. In these latter cases, there was simply not enough space on the farms to keep them. Sometimes there was a limited amount of feed. As time went by, dairy cows needed to go out to grass, and would need to be moved from farm to field and back again, twice daily. Suddenly, from having no farm calls to make, we had the huge task of undertaking 'pre-movement inspections'. This meant that we had to visit and inspect any animals before they were moved from a farm to go directly to slaughter. We were also given the task of issuing licences to move animals from farm to farm under special circumstances. This became the activity that took most of our day and we became experts in inspection and, more importantly, the filling in of paperwork.

On a typical day, at this point in the outbreak, I would do

between ten and twenty movement inspection visits. About twenty minutes would be spent inspecting the animals for signs of suspicious disease, followed by about thirty minutes filling in and processing the paperwork. As the disease got closer and closer to Thirsk, I noticed that the time needed to do the paperwork seemed to become greater, which left us with less time to inspect the animals. This was ironic, as we should really have been focusing more time on the inspection rather than the forms. We simply did not have enough hours in the day. Pigs would be loaded, in the darkness, for movement to slaughter at 5 a.m. most mornings, so this was the start of our day. I'm not sure quite how effective our bleary-eyed inspections were at this time, but nevertheless, everybody was relieved once the all-important piece of paper was handed over. We would go on like this all day, and I remember arriving on one farm at 10.30 in the evening to undertake the last inspection of the day by torchlight. If anything suspicious was identified it spelt disaster for the farmer, and his neighbours. The pigs or cattle would not be able to be moved, and draconian restrictions would be placed. Panic would ensue, and MAFF vets would swoop in with their conspicuous white overalls.

In these early stages of the epidemic, the other type of inspection in our area was the 'Dangerous Contact Tracing Visit'. These were undertaken by MAFF vets, or vets who had been recruited by MAFF to help with the outbreak. They involved inspecting farms where there were considered to be animals at risk, for example, cattle or sheep that had been at the same market as an infected animal. MAFF produced elegant maps criss-crossed with lines tracing the progress of those animals known to have been infected. Dangerous Contact Tracing Visits were conspicuous, because unfamiliar vehicles would be spotted at the end of a farm track and men in white plastic suits would be seen squirting their boots with disinfectant. One particular veterinary inspector, who had been coerced out of retirement to help with these inspections, was more conspicuous that most. He drove a Rolls-Royce with the personalized number plate VET. I never met him, but I had seen his vehicle and his large frame, wrapped in white plastic, from a distance. Wherever his car was seen, rumours would follow. Suspicion and stories were everywhere and rumours of cases – lame sheep seen in fields, for example – spread quickly through the close-knit and terrified community.

On one occasion there was great consternation that there had been a confirmed case just up the road, about half a mile from our practice. A collection of vehicles had been spotted in the layby, outside Mile House Farm on the road to York. Several people, all dressed in white outfits, were congregating with intent, and by lunchtime it seemed certain that Mr Swales' farm had 'gone down with it'. Only later did the truth emerge. Thirsk's crown green bowling team had an away fixture at York that day, and the team had agreed to meet in the layby so they could all share a lift together. Apparently the competition gear for crown green bowling is an all-white outfit.

By the end of the first few weeks of the outbreak, the nearest case or 'infected premises' as MAFF quaintly called the affected farms, was about 15 miles north of Thirsk in the village of Picton. It was not a farm to which we attended, and it was sufficiently isolated from most of our other farms that we felt reasonably safe. We had weathered the early part of the foot-and-mouth storm. Other parts of North Yorkshire, especially Wensleydale and, later, the upper parts of Wharfedale, were being decimated by the rampaging disease. The first case on a farm that I actually knew was in Threshfield near Grassington. By this point, MAFFs website was up and running and we could see all the new outbreaks. It was a family farm where I had spent several happy and informative weeks as a young and enthusiastic student. I knew how devastated they would be, and I sent them a card extending my sympathies. Admittedly it was not much help, but I felt I had, somehow, to acknowledge the terrible time they were going through.

Other parts of the country were being ravaged too, and the farming community was in a state of perpetual fear. Two of our friends, Cath, with whom I shared a house at vet school, and her fiancé Andy, a dairy farmer, were due to get married. They lived near Gloucester, but Cath was from Scotland and their wedding was to take place in the small village of Rannoch in the Highlands. There was much concern about a hundred guests, nearly all vets and dairy farmers, descending on this little village in an area which, so far, was free from foot-and-mouth. It looked as if the wedding might have to be called off. Not only were the residents of Rannoch afraid, but farmers were reluctant to travel at all, for fear of spread of the disease. However, after much debate, it was decided that the celebration could go ahead, provided we all thoroughly scrubbed and disinfected our cars before leaving home. I kept an eye on MAFF's website to check if there had been any suspect cases cropping up in the Highlands for weeks after our visit.

The practice had an elderly lady client who was very sprightly but slightly eccentric. Mrs G lived in a small village surrounded by cattle and sheep, on the hills above Thirsk. Her family's farm was one of the closest in the practice to the Picton case, and I would get regular updates of the situation in her village. One evening, I returned from an early season cricket match, to a slightly bemused Anne, who had taken a very cryptic message from Mrs G. The conversation had gone something like this:

'Hello, can I speak with Julian, please?'

'I'm afraid he's not in. Can I take a message?'

'Where is he?'

'He's playing cricket at Ampleforth.'

'Oh. Can you tell him to phone me after dark?'

'Yes. I'll ask him to give you a ring when he gets back.'

'No. Please tell Julian to phone me *after dark*.'

So, after I got back from cricket, I waited until darkness had fallen, then returned the call.

Mrs G had information about lorries passing her house and through her village. It was unusual because the village was small, and lorries did not often frequent the tiny lanes. She was suspicious that the vehicles were being used to transport dead animals – something that had been happening in affected areas, as animals were killed on the farm and then loaded up to be taken to the nearest pyre. It was causing general concern, and rightly so, that this could be a source of spread of the disease. She wanted to know if there had been a case nearby? I think the significance of the darkness was so that she wasn't seen through her window passing on sensitive information, although I'm still not sure! On that occasion there was no such case near her village, but it wasn't long before our first farm was flagged up to be culled as a 'dangerous contact'. It had only been a matter of time.

It was another evening telephone call, this time from a farmer who had cattle, sheep and pigs. His was my favourite farm to visit.

'They want to come and kill everything tomorrow morning,' was John's typically phlegmatic opening sentence. 'What can we do?'

John and I had been friends ever since I first started at the practice, and I got on very well with him and all of his staff. Tom and Ray were two of the best stockmen I have ever worked with and it was always a great pleasure to tend to their animals. Soon after I started work at Thirsk, I had diagnosed an insidious disease called bovine viral diarrhoea, or BVD, in his herd. There had been subtle but serious problems with the herd over quite some time, and when the diagnosis was made, John's mother, who was one of those dynamic elderly ladies with undying enthusiasm, knowledge and vigour, arranged a meeting with John, myself, Ray and Tom to discuss how to tackle the disease. This kind of herd planning is now commonplace in large animal veterinary practice, but at that time it was a very forward-thinking step. As a new vet it was a daunting meeting, but as a result, we developed a great and friendly working relationship and mutual respect. So it was a sad day, that June evening, when I got that phone call. A neighbouring farm had had its animals killed under the 'Slaughter on Suspicion' rule, that meant animals could be killed before laboratory tests had confirmed the presence of foot-and-mouth. It was a contentious policy but was seen as crucial, to avoid the delay of four days it took for the laboratory to achieve a definitive diagnosis. It was argued that this four-day wait could allow further spread. John's farm was within one and a half kilometres of this

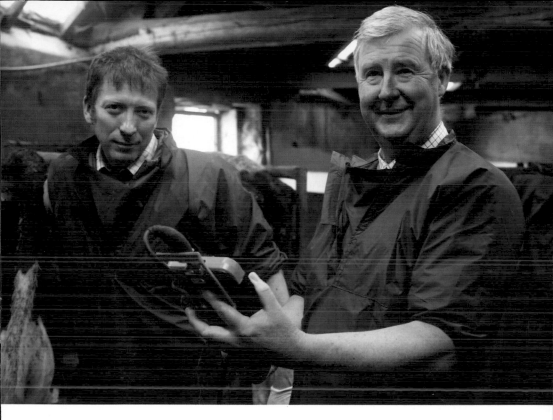

Above: With my friend and colleague Peter Wright in an early publicity photograph for *The Yorkshire Vet* TV series. (*Daisybeck Studios/GroupM Entertainment/Channel 5*)

Below: Examining a litter of pups is always a high point in our busy days. This is a very cute litter of Shih Tzu puppies. (*Daisybeck Studios/GroupM Entertainment/Channel 5*)

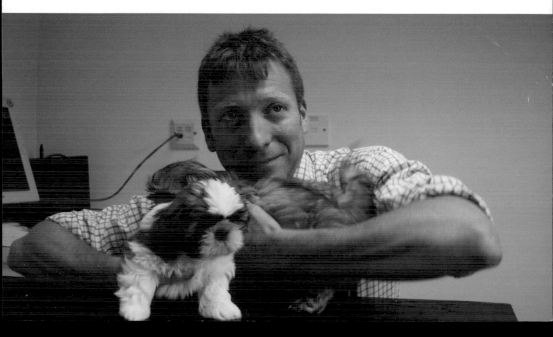

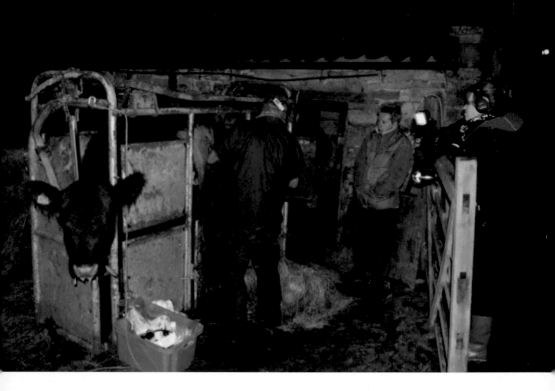

Above and below: Performing a caesarean on a heifer at two o'clock on a bitterly cold morning, as producer-director Laura Blair, dressed in many layers of clothes, films every detail from a safe vantage point. It never ceases to amaze me how well our farm-animal patients will tolerate what they are sometimes subjected to. The heifer made a full recovery.

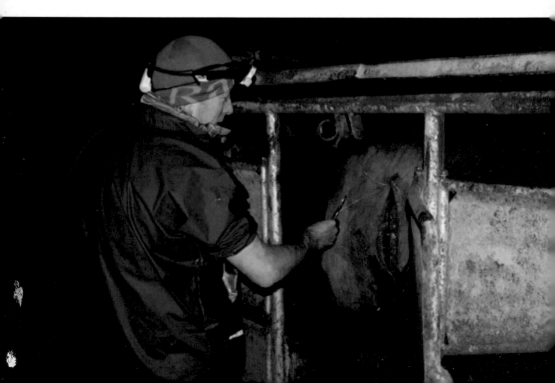

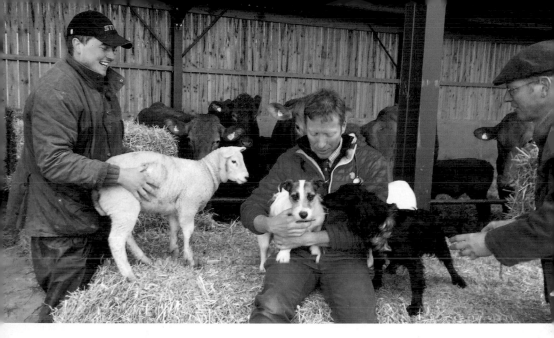

Above: A moment to compare our animals. The Bell family are, quite rightly, proud of their beautiful stock, but surely my faithful Jack Russell terrier, Emmy, is the cutest?

Below: Paul and Jane Blanchard with their pygmy goat. This one had a skin condition caused by a mite infestation. She was pretty scabby and sore, but responded well to the treatment. David fastidiously captures it all. (*Daisybeck Studios/GroupM Entertainment/Channel 5*)

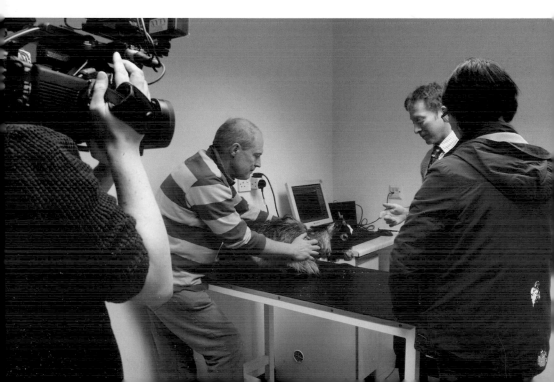

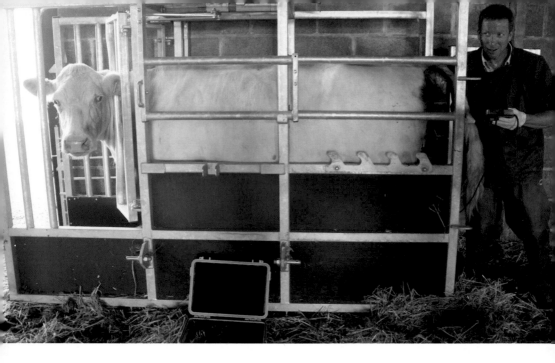

Above: Pregnancy testing a Whitebred Shorthorn cow. This is a standard part of our job and much of the time of a large animal vet is spent – literally – with his arm inside a cow's backside.

Below: Examining the testicles of a stock bull forms part of a pre-breeding examination. When squatting behind a bull, close to his back legs and directly under his tail, the risks are obvious!

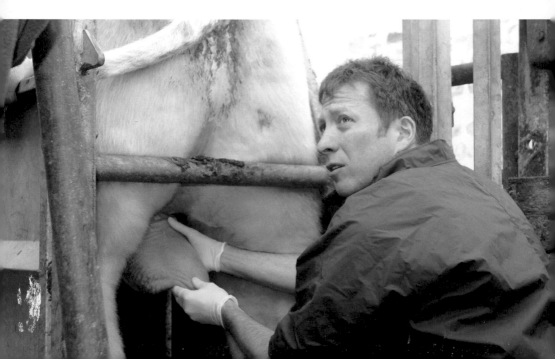

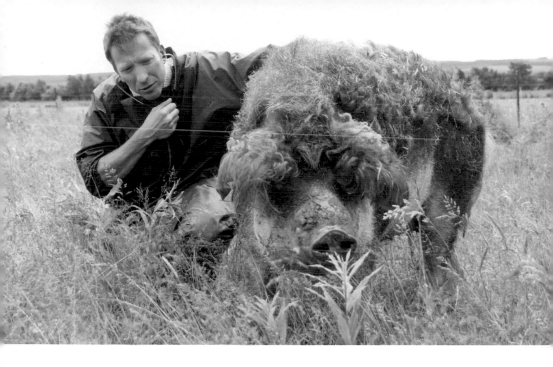

Above: Attempting to examine a pig – always a difficult task! Mangalitsa pigs are very unusual and covered in thick, woolly hair – and often have a mind of their own.

Below: Farmer Lisa loves her pigs! They are not always as friendly as this. Her partner, standing out of shot, has a large and clumsy bandage on his right hand where his tendons have been lacerated by the tusks of an uncooperative sow.

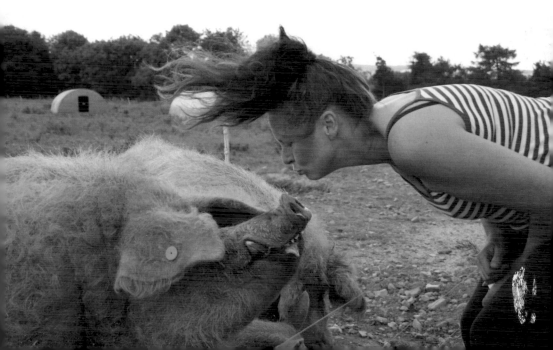

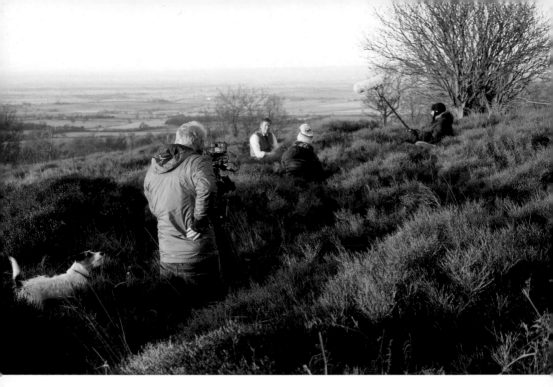

Above: Filming shots for the opening titles of *The Yorkshire Vet* above the White Horse of Kilburn. I persuaded the team we should meet at six a.m., the light was wonderful as the sun rose. (*Daisybeck Studios/GroupM Entertainment/Channel 5*)

Below: Visiting the Great Yorkshire Show with Peter. We rarely get the chance to have an afternoon out together, even less so to look at healthy animals in top condition in the show ring. Izzy never missed a chance to capture these moments on film.

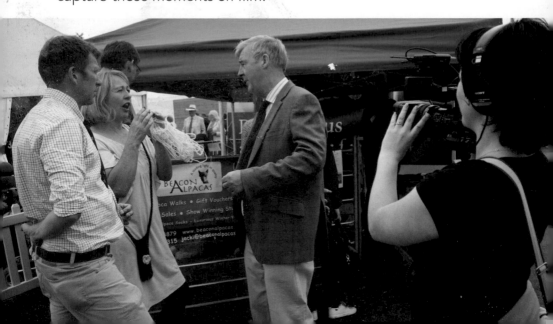

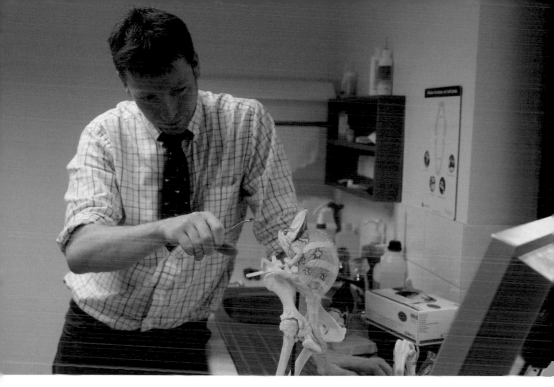

Above: One of our more unusual patients – a chameleon: sitting here on the plastic model of a dog's pelvis. (*Daisybeck Studios/GroupM Entertainment/Channel 5*)

Below: Another nighttime call. This poor dog had inhaled a barley head and was coughing up blood. The seed head was very difficult to remove as it was lodged at the bottom of his lungs. It was painstaking work with my endoscope. (*Daisybeck Studios/GroupM Entertainment/Channel 5*)

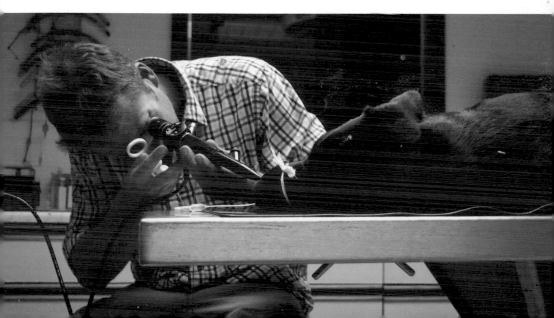

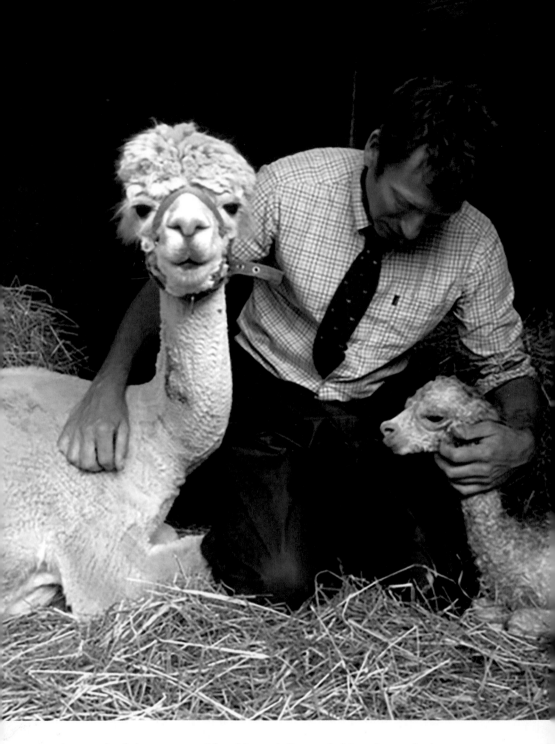

A wonderful moment: I had just delivered this cria – a baby alpaca – after a very challenging 'breech' birth. I had to carefully unravel and unfold its (very long) legs to allow its safe delivery. Baby is sitting up already and mum looks relieved, if slightly bemused!

suspected case, and his animals were therefore subject to being killed under the equally contentious 'Contiguous Cull' policy. This was a policy introduced to kill animals on farms surrounding a confirmed or suspected case. There was, apparently, a one in three chance that animals within a one and a half kilometre radius would contract the disease. Therefore killing them immediately would (in theory) stop its onward spread.

I cancelled my evening arrangements and immediately set about getting all the facts, or as many as I could, about the nearby case, the whereabouts of John's animals, proximity to roads and other barriers to disease transmission such as woods, arable fields or rivers. It became clear that his pigs were the animals most at risk, as they were closest to the IP (infected premises). The rest of his animals were grazing several kilometres away on the opposite side of a major dual carriageway. They were isolated from any other stock to the east by woodland and moors, and therefore clearly no risk to any other farms. The obvious and sensible plan was to cull the pigs and monitor the rest of the animals for signs of disease. Pigs were a major risk in the spread of disease because they shed vastly more virus than other animals, so in the face of this suspected outbreak, they really did need to be culled. However, it seemed clear that there was absolutely no need to kill the other healthy cattle and sheep, which were well out of the risk zone.

My protests to the duty officer at the Newcastle Animal Health office fell on deaf ears. MAFF's killing spree was in full flow by now, and no one was going to listen to the sensible objections of a vet on the ground, even though he might actually have some useful information and comment to make. Policy was dogmatic, unwavering and, sadly, misguided in many ways.

Thankfully, we were not involved in the killing on IPs.

This intrusion onto our first farm focused everybody's thoughts in the area. Until now, Thirsk had been reasonably unaffected by clinical cases and restrictions on normal life were based on the pre-movement rules and inspections, the increasing numbers of tracing checks and things like footpath closures (which appeared to be blanket, regardless of whether footpaths went anywhere near grazing animals). But now everything had changed. Disinfectant mats and footbaths appeared everywhere and paranoia descended. One farmer sold his Land Rover and swapped it for a car, because he thought it would be easier to disinfect. Another took to his bicycle as a means of transport for the same reasons, though this turned out to be futile as his farm eventually succumbed to the disease.

One evening, Anne was returning home across the A66, after visiting her aunt in Lancashire. It was mainly single carriageway, so it was difficult to overtake lorries and, as often happened, she was stuck behind one. She was alarmed to see a noxious liquid dribbling out of the back of the lorry and all over the road. Not just all over the road, but all over her car. When she tried to use her windscreen wipers to clears the splashes that were obscuring her view, horrible fatty grease was smeared all over the windscreen. Eventually when the chance arose to overtake, it was obvious that the lorry was of the kind that Mrs G had spotted going through her village. It was one of the lorries that carried culled foot and mouth-infected animals to a burial site, rendering facility or pyre. It was leaking infected fluid all over one of the main roads across the north of the country. Was there any wonder we could not control this highly infectious disease? Anne detoured on her journey back home, through a car wash and disinfection point. With this kind of grotesque and clumsy error, what on earth was the point in selling your Land Rover and travelling around Thirsk on your bicycle?

Increasingly, as the epidemic progressed, there was growing cynicism about the management and handling of it. Episodes such as this added to the speculation that the spread of the disease was being perpetuated by the killing teams. They had much to gain financially, as the slaughter teams, disinfectant teams and transportation companies had negotiated lucrative contracts to provide their services on an immediate and urgent basis. One farmer whose cows became infected with the disease found the tail of a cow in the same field in which he first saw signs in his own animals. He drew the obvious conclusions. Vets swarmed from all corners of the world to work for MAFF. The South Africans, in particular, did well. The value of the rand against the pound meant that South African vets could earn the equivalent of three years' salary in just six months. Foot-and-mouth disease was prevalent in South Africa, and they really didn't see what all the excitement was about.

There were allegations that some farmers actually *wanted* the disease to be confirmed on their farms, or were *trying* to become condemned as dangerous contacts, as the financial compensation for compulsory slaughter of your herd or flock was, quite rightly, substantial. Certainly, it could be considered that an elderly farmer, on the point of retirement and disillusioned with farming, could not get a better end-of-career payout, just like the mining redundancies for coal miners in the 1980s. However, I have to say, I did not see this at all, and when the disease finally hit Thirsk, not one farmer I met nor anyone connected with the industry had this sentiment. Generally, people who farm stock care deeply about that stock and it is, more often than not, their life's work. In fact, when foot-and-mouth struck Thirsk, I have rarely seen men, young and old, as broken.

Cynicism was also hanging over the government's handling of the outbreak, and its motives became increasingly under scrutiny. Allegedly, some compensation cheques were signed by the 'European Stock Reduction Fund', suggesting that there was a plan behind the extensive and wanton killing, over and above the desire to halt the spread of disease. There were rumours that MAFF had ordered huge supplies of wooden railway sleepers just weeks before the outbreak started. Apparently, this was attributed to a strategic planning exercise being undertaken by MAFF that happened to be scheduled immediately before the disease appeared. Who would have thought the department was as well organized as that? At this point, super-efficient organization did not seem its forte and so the speculation was, rightly or wrongly, that it had been buying up wood for the enormous pyres, and its credibility was questioned still further.

And, of course, what about vaccination?

Both human and veterinary medicine has benefited from this wonderful tool in the battle against infectious disease. Discovered in the late eighteenth century and refined by Edward Jenner, the first vaccine for a human disease – smallpox – was developed from a similar contagious disease of cattle – cowpox. The irony that cows had been inextricably connected with the discovery and refinement of the process of vaccination is inescapable. Nearly two hundred years later, rather than benefiting from the biotechnology that would have saved tens of thousands of animals, cattle and sheep were not privileged enough to make use of this preventative technique. It was deemed, in the UK, that the best way to prevent an animal getting a disease was to kill it. Of course, the reasons for not using vaccination were down to compliance with EU rules and also its impact on the trade of our livestock and its meat with the rest of the world. It seemed to escape the notice of the politicians that, if the killing continued as it was, we simply wouldn't have any livestock to export anyway. Despite avoiding vaccination, the country was still banned from exporting meat and live animals for a year, because the UK was a country that had actually had the disease. The Netherlands, by contrast, swiftly used vaccination in the very early outbreaks that occurred there, in the spring of 2001. Their epidemic, using vaccination as a control method, lasted only two months. I do not know of a European country whose meat export industry is more critical to its economy than that of the Netherlands. The Netherlands exports five times as much beef as the UK and a many times greater volume of pork. This country had an altogether different way of handling the outbreak to *preserve* its export industry. The inflexible EU rules were treated much more flexibly on their side of the channel.

However, as things stood, we were stuck in the middle of an epidemic, and to object to the process or to the decisions of the government and MAFF was futile. As far as I remember there was little objection raised by the various veterinary bodies at the time, and we all simply complied with the dogmatic rules. There was nothing to be gained by an individual stance. The steamroller was too big and it was fully steamed up.

14

Life in the Protection Zone

Inevitably, it happened – a clinical case on one of our farms. It was in an idyllic spot just outside the village of Knayton. The farm was a lovely place, a traditional suckler herd with gentle, Hereford cross cows and the most kind and gentle stockman called Bert.

I was at Thirsk auction mart, inspecting all the cattle and sheep as they went through the market. I had been there since 5 a.m., and I was, yet again, bleary eyed. I was also on duty, so I had my beeper and phone with me, as I worked my way through the sheep, checking mouth after mouth for the telltale signs of blistering or ulcers, and watched every cow for signs of limping and excessive salivation. There were no signs to be seen this morning. At least, nothing at the auction mart. But, at 7.30 my beeper went off with a message asking me to phone the farmer, this time not after dark but immediately. Bert had been out to check his cattle as they grazed in their field, first thing this Thursday morning. They were all standing still and would not come up to the feed trough to eat. Worse still, they were all drooling heavily. What should he do? I felt sick. There was little doubt that the animals had foot-and-mouth disease. I knew I couldn't go myself to see the cattle. I still had a lot of animals to examine at the auction mart, and if I attended an infected premises, I would be unable to leave until MAFF had gone through all their procedures. I would also not be allowed to see any farm animals for a week afterwards, to avoid further spread. I gave Bert instructions to phone MAFF and give them all the details directly.

His animals were dead within the day and everything in Thirsk stopped. I knew I would not be supervizing the sale of animals at Thirsk auction mart for some time. All movements were stopped and, since this farm was slap bang in the middle of our area, most of the practice catchment was in the so-called 'protection zone'. This meant all animals needed to be inspected every forty-eight hours. The cattle and sheep movement inspections that we had arranged that day were suspended, and we held our breath.

It was the first week of July 2001. By this stage, there were about twenty to thirty new cases of foot and mouth occurring every day across the country, compared with just short of three hundred per day in March, when the disease was at its height. This meant that most of the country, and the media in particular, had lost interest, but for us in Thirsk, the nightmare was just beginning. As the media and government were declaring 'the countryside open', our villages had culling teams and disinfectant tankers parked all over their grass verges. The killing spree on our farms was truly horrific. The worst point was the day my good friend, Jonathon, the guy who had swapped his car for a bike to try to reduce the risk of infection, found signs in his herd. He was the same age as me, and as I bought into the partnership at the practice, he was taking over the reins of the farm from his father. His milking cows were very dear to him and, of everyone I knew, he was the most tangibly traumatized by the devastation. The day his cows were being killed, I drove to the top of Sutton Bank and went for a walk along the footpath above Gormire, a beautiful lake nestling below the dramatic limestone cliff. Alf Wight referred to this view as 'the finest view in England'. He was right most of the time, but not on this day. A murky, humid mist hung in the air and there was no wind at all. Eerily, there was no noise either, other than the regular banging of the guns of the cull team, and the hollow moos of cattle being rounded up against their will.

I was seeking solitude and time to rationalize what was happening, but before long I bumped into another farmer called Clive, who had sheep and cattle in a village about a mile away, hopefully safe, at the top of the bank. He was pulling heavily on his hand-rolled cigarettes and I thought about asking him for one, such was my state. We couldn't really think of anything to say to one another, so we stood there for a few moments and then just walked on, in our own separate directions. It was strange, but there was no need for words.

The closest I came to seeing the disease first hand was during a routine inspection on a large herd of beef cattle. By now, all cattle and sheep in the protection zone (essentially, all our farms) needed to be checked for signs of disease, by a vet, every forty-eight hours. The owner of this particular farm was insistent that MAFF vets did not set foot on his premises, given all the suspicion that MAFF officials were actually, inadvertently, spreading the disease themselves since they had been onto so many infected premises. MAFF, somewhat reluctantly, agreed to let us do some of these checks and I went to the farm every two days for about a month, in my lunch break. The phrase 'lunch break' was tenuous, as I hadn't had a break at lunchtime for months. The cattle were all at grass, so the farmer left me the keys to his quad bike and I would drive around, looking at them all as they grazed in the fields. Aside from being dressed from head to toe in plastic in the heat of the day, it was quite a pleasant way to spend an hour. I could drive up to the cattle and watch them quietly eating grass, and it felt a little bit like being on safari. The cattle were large, traditional and beautiful and it was a great chance to see them contented and in their natural setting. Mostly when we see cattle they are corralled into a handling pen or they are sick and in need of treatment. These cattle were happy and healthy, although as I watched them I was also aware of the tiny specks of men in white suits on the hillside above the farm. I knew those particular white suits did not belong to Thirsk crown green bowling club. The disease was nearby and I had to be vigilant.

I could easily assess the health of the cattle as they grazed in their fields, as sick animals would not walk or eat – instead, they would drool heavily, just like the Herefords near Knayton. However, the next time I visited, on a Friday, I asked the stockman to bring some of the cows in, so I could inspect their mouths and feet in more detail. I usually did this on every second visit or if there was anything suspicious. I arrived, as usual, at lunchtime, but it was not until half past nine in the evening that I left, dressed only in my pants and drenched in disinfectant, with my clothes sealed in a plastic bin bag. I thought I had encountered foot-and-mouth disease first hand and I was very worried.

I had gathered a bunch of about thirty young cattle in the collecting yard and observed. It was hard to say they were actually poorly, but they didn't look quite right. Many had thin drools of mucousy saliva dribbling from the corner of their mouths. The more I looked, the more I noticed problems. Many of the calves were shifting their weight from foot to foot, as if they had hot feet. On closer inspection the top of the hooves, around the coronary band, was reddish pink and looked sore. I put each of them in the crush for closer inspection. About a third had superficial and small erosions on their gums. I could see no actual ulcers in their mouths – the hallmark of foot-and-mouth – and no actual lesions on the feet. Most of the cattle had temperatures elevated to around 103 degrees Fahrenheit. This was high, but not the 104 or 105 degrees that was symptomatic of the viral infection. The cows seemed to be healthier than the calves, but we were worried. Neither of us had seen anything like this before. It wasn't classic foot-and-mouth, but it was worrying enough to make the call to MAFF – sick-looking cattle, high temperatures, mouth lesions, drooling, sore feet, within a protection zone and within sight of men in white suits. The veterinary officer on the end of the telephone was less than helpful, and his tone of voice was not what I was expecting.

'Are you one of us?' was his first question. Initially, I didn't understand what he meant by this. In what way? A fellow colleague, or a fellow human being? It soon became clear that he meant a fellow MAFF vet.

I explained that I wasn't a MAFF vet, but a private practitioner, working on behalf of MAFF, to inspect cattle within a protection zone at the request of the farmer. At this, he seemed even less convinced about my assessment of the situation. He considered 103 degrees Fahrenheit to be a normal temperature for a calf. I wondered when he had last seen and treated an actual animal. Our conversation was tense, but eventually he agreed to send two MAFF vets to give their verdict, and gave me permission to leave the farm, suitably disinfected, once they had arrived. The two Australian vets who appeared late that evening had both seen clinical cases before. To their credit, they phoned me at home to give me their assessment – another telephone call 'after dark'. In short, they couldn't decide, so planned to re-examine the cattle, early the following morning, to see how the clinical signs had progressed. This seemed a sensible course of action, as genuine foot-and-mouth would undoubtedly have advanced to the point where a diagnosis was much more clear, twelve hours later.

I did not hear from the Australian vets again, but I anxiously telephoned the farmer the following morning, a Saturday, to find out the news.

'We're all clear,' was the excited reply.

'OK, great. What now?' I assumed that tests had been taken and sent off to the lab for confirmation of the negative diagnosis and, just as important, to find out the actual cause of the signs. If it wasn't foot-and-mouth, what was it? To me this was the next obvious question.

As it transpired, samples had been taken of some cattle, but once the pronouncement of a negative diagnosis had been made, these were discarded, and not allowed to leave the farm (it was on a 'D' notice, which meant animals, manure, samples and so on could not leave). I continued my inspections every forty-eight hours for the next few weeks and saw no more signs of disease. I wanted to take samples to check for other causes of mouth lesions that might explain the problems, but I was thwarted again. Ironically, it was impossible to test for foot-and-mouth since this would trigger the farm being reclassified as a suspect case and the animals would be killed as a 'Slaughter on Suspicion' – a classic 'catch-22'. Several months later, when everything had settled down, I revisited the farm and took several blood tests from cattle that had been drooling, with sore mouths. I sent them to the lab to check for other diseases that may have been the cause of the problems. Every test came back negative. The obvious next question was: 'Was this foot-and-mouth disease after all?' There is now no way of knowing, but I remain convinced that it was indeed the virus. My theory is, that in this old, established and traditional breed of cow, possibly with some inherent resistant to the virus, foot-and-mouth had not manifested itself in the same virulent manner that it did in more vulnerable and genetically frail dairy cows. The herd survived and lives on. I'm going there next week to do some jobs. It was a lucky herd and luckier than most at that time in Thirsk.

The pattern of spread was quite surprising and hard to predict in our area. The disease followed, in part, the contours of the Hambleton Hills, from north to south, but like many unfit cyclists, it didn't make it up Sutton Bank, and no confirmed cases appeared to the east of this escarpment. After the village of Thirlby, it stopped its progress following the curve of the hills, and went south towards the Vale of York. There was much worry that it might affect the pig farms of East Yorkshire. Pigs apparently sent large plumes of virus spiralling in all directions and, according to MAFF, if they were infected the disease would go wild. We thought it had already gone wild as there were very few farms left with any stock. Nevertheless, the enthusiastic killing continued and most of the farms up to a small village called Bagby, one mile from the practice, lost all their animals. Then, in the middle of August, it suddenly stopped. There was a large tract of arable land to the south of Bagby, but this didn't seem fully to explain the halt. It was almost as if the outbreak got bored and ran out of steam.

So now, six months after the first case, it seemed the crisis was over. At least it was for the farmers. They now had many months of cleaning and disinfection to do. Their farms had never been so clean. Or so empty. During this time, as the vets who attended their needs, we had nearly no farm work to do. On a personal level, I had only recently bought into the practice and now we had lost over half of our farm clients. We had had no income from this side of our practice for nearly a year. How many farms would restock? We guessed some would, but not all. What would they restock with? One farmer, who had two large dairy herds and a massive pig enterprise, spent his compensation on large tracts of housing. This was probably a sensible and lucrative move, but not very helpful for a young vet hoping to pay off his business loan. Eventually the empty farms had 'sentinel' sheep added to them, which were blood tested at intervals to see if they had developed antibodies to the disease. This would confirm or rule out the persistent presence of the virus on the unit, and hopefully confirm the thoroughness of the disinfection regime. We had hoped that this blood testing might provide the practice with a role and some income, but this was not to be either. Blood testing a handful of sheep was a great little job for older vets on the cusp of retirement and they snapped up the work. As it happened, some farms did return to livestock, but for many it was an opportune time to leave the crumbling industry. After the BSE crisis ten years earlier, followed by this catastrophic episode, it was a miracle that the UK still had a livestock industry at all. After this chapter, it was severely battered and that had knock-on effects to everyone connected to it. Most of the farms that did restock, did so in a different way. One large dairy herd nearby had farmed two hundred head of dairy cattle but restocked with about forty alpacas. While this is a great diversification and a much easier lifestyle than milking cows twice a day, it doesn't provide much work for the local vet, tanker driver or foot trimmer, or give many sales to the local feed merchant. The fabric of our rural economy had changed irreversibly.

The practice had survived but we all, individually, had emerged emotionally drained, tired and extremely stressed by the whole experience. On a personal level, I had been left with a persistent and lingering dermatitis, which I put down to a reaction to the copious amounts of disinfectant that I had been using. However, even after our use of the iodine-based solutions had decreased to pre-epidemic levels, the persistent itchy lesions on my back stubbornly refused to go away.

15

The Persistent Itch

I had spent a large part of 2001 enveloped in a plastic outfit and doused with iodine, as part of the effort to reduce the risk of spreading foot-and-mouth disease. As vets, we always clean and disinfect our boots before leaving a farm, but in 2001 we took this to epic proportions, and would spend tracts of time every day cleaning and spraying ourselves, and our vehicles, with disinfectant. After visits we would literally cover ourselves in the stuff. The smell was everywhere. This, coupled with the sweaty environment inside my plastic overalls, could easily explain the itchy lesions that appeared all over my back. I'd never suffered from this problem before, but after constant sleepless nights spent scratching to the point of bleeding, and after several failed attempts with veterinary remedies (well, they work in dogs, so I guessed they would be good for me!), I went to see the doctor, who thought it was eczema. I was sent away with large tubs of cream, similar in appearance to the 'evil salve'. The cream was as ineffective as my own veterinary treatments.

It took many more GP visits, and various homegrown attempts at diagnosis and treatment (including going out in the middle of the night to the newly opened twenty-four-hour Tesco to buy a complete new set of clothes, in case it was caused by an allergy to the washing powder we used), before I was referred to the dermatologist. After a six-week wait (I manage to see *my* itchy patients the same day), I visited the specialist at Friarage Hospital in Northallerton. I owe much to this man for, despite taking multiple calls on his mobile phone during the consultation, he knew instantly the cause of my intractable itchiness. I went for a biopsy (another month's wait: I biopsy my skin cases the next day), which confirmed the diagnosis. Far from being eczema or an allergy to disinfectant, I had a condition called dermatitis herpetiformis.

Dermatitis herpetiformis is a rare skin manifestation of coeliac disease and is caused by intolerance to gluten. According to one internet forum, the extreme discomfort it brings is described as follows: 'You get completely sunburnt, fall in a patch of nettles and then jump in an ants' nest.' It is so desperately itchy and so under-diagnosed by doctors that some sufferers commit suicide. I felt lucky to have had a relatively early diagnosis. Not that I was ever quite at the point of suicide, but I was in a pretty desperate place. During those months in 2001, I had been faced with the anxiety of foot-and-mouth disease and the stress of not knowing whether my newly purchased business would have a future without cattle and sheep. I had survived on precious little sleep because of the terrible itchiness and, on top of this, the industrial doses of antihistamines that I had been prescribed, when it was assumed to be an allergy, meant that every time I sat down on a sofa, I fell asleep. My energy levels were at an all-time low and my pasty complexion was clue enough to my perilously low iron levels, also caused by the disease. Clients would often comment about me looking tired, and I knew there had also been a handful of comments about me not being very cheerful during consultations. The diagnosis of DH, although very serious, at least provided some explanation for my pallor, itchiness and general weariness. Thinking back, I saw that the signs had been present for longer than I had realized. It explained why, after excelling at cross country at school, I lost all my speed and form, and never rose above the fourth team in the university cross country club, when really I should easily have been able to make the second team. The undergraduate's diet of toast, pies, pasta and beer could not have been more packed with gluten. I could not have designed a more toxic diet if I had tried.

I had always regarded myself as somewhat invincible and able to tackle any physical task, whether it was dehorning twenty cows, working all night on call, running the Three Peaks fell race or cycling to Everest base camp. However, now it seemed that I was, in fact, utterly and completely vulnerable and my health was in ruins. I had discovered my very own kryptonite. All it would take to make me sick and weak was one crumb of pork pie or one bite of a bread roll.

Despite being buoyed by finally having a diagnosis, and with it the possibility of managing the condition, I was not completely delighted to hear my fate. Itchy skin and general fatigue apart, dermatitis herpetiformis confers on its sufferers a massively increased risk of succumbing to a whole list of other serious diseases. Leukaemia, thyroid disorders and rheumatoid arthritis are high on the list. I knew about these conditions because my four-legged patients could be affected by the same problems. Not only would I have DH for the rest of my life, but I was now absolutely certain I would get one of these other horrible conditions. Apart from all that, how on earth would I manage without a pint? (Beer was full of gluten, so that was off the list.) This was surely the time when I needed one more than ever.

But: 'Good news!' the dermatologist told me. There was medication that would alleviate all the signs of this disease. I needed to take it, on top of my restricted diet. It was called dapsone. We had learnt about dapsone in pharmacology lectures with the medics at college, as its main use was in the treatment of leprosy. At least this meant that the tips of my fingers would be in robust health, I thought. It is nasty stuff, though. I needed regular blood tests to check my red cell count, since my blood cells could easily be destroyed by the drug. My liver enzymes and various other parameters also had to be looked at. At the start, I was being monitored more regularly than my chemotherapy patients. The list of side effects, which were genuine rather than simply written on the data sheet for caution, was startling, and extended as far as mental disturbances, and possible psychosis.

Despite all the negative connotations of my condition, new diet, and potentially toxic medication, I knew that making important changes to my lifestyle would result in a very healthy me again, and I embraced the start of a new era. I was extremely fortunate to have had DH flagged up so promptly. During my research into the disease, I learnt that the signs are greatly exacerbated by exposure to high levels of iodine. This explained why it came on so severely during the foot-and-mouth crisis. Had I not been so completely marinated in iodine over this period it might never have been identified.

The improvement in my symptoms on starting my leprosy medicine was immediate and dramatic. The itching stopped pretty much straightaway and the blisters started to heal. Once I had familiarized myself with my new diet, I began to feel much better and fitter. Nowadays gluten-free foods are readily available and do not carry the same freakish stigma of weak, pale hypochondriacs that they did then. Back in 2002 the bread was the size, taste and consistency of a beer mat, with an aftertaste of vinegar. Gluten-free pasta would instantly turn to gloopy soup and gluten-free flour, appetizingly referred to as 'white mix', was more like powdered Polyfilla. These gluten-free substitutes were not really worth exploring. The weekly Tesco shopping trip took on a whole new complicated twist, as every label and packet had to be scrutinized. Anne, who wasn't the most enthusiastic of cooks at the best of times, took on the challenge of trying to do some gluten-free baking. She resorted to phoning her mother in Hampshire, to get her to make the same thing, so she could tell if it was her cooking skills or the gluten-free ingredients that had caused the strange appearance of her latest endeavour. The upside of this was that the successful outcomes in Hampshire would appear a few days later, parcelled up, brought by a postman who was weighed down with double-density loaves.

On a holiday to France with some friends, soon after my diagnosis in the summer of 2002, I hadn't really quite got to grips with my new dietary constraints. While everyone else tucked into baguettes and cheese at lunchtime, I would eat half a Camembert and a tomato – not the most balanced of diets. However, once I got used to it, I quickly realized that a diet naturally free of gluten was, as long as I excluded neat cheese, a very healthy one. Rice, potatoes, fruit, vegetables, fish and meat, yoghurt, nuts, honey, wine and gin and tonic – it was a great combination and a mixture on which I now thrive. No biscuits, pies, buns or beer. I would urge anyone to give it a go. I do have to be incredibly strict though, because even the smallest crumb in the butter dish or half a teaspoon of wheat flour in a sauce or gravy will mess everything up. If I accidentally eat even the tiniest trace of gluten, it takes me about three weeks to return to normal and my immune system, apparently, takes months to recover.

———

At the time of our French holiday, Anne was pregnant, so the Camembert was off the menu for her, as well as the French wine (all in all, it was not a great choice of holiday destinations, under the circumstances). The DH was coming under control, life in Thirsk was gradually returning to some sort of normality and we were embracing the idea of bringing new life into our world. Anne was due to give birth the following January. This would surely be straightforward, we thought, as we knew all about animals. Surely a small baby is just like a young puppy, lamb or calf? We took the first ultrasound scan in our stride. We were used to looking at scans so it was no great revelation.

The same could not be said for Linda, a friend and client who had been coming to see me for several years with her cat, Toby. Toby was suffering from terrible gingivitis. It was painful and intractable, and the result of the body's own immune system attacking the gum tissue, leading to an awful bleeding inflammation that made it almost impossible for Toby to eat. Some cats with this condition actually hiss at their food, as if blaming the food for the pain. Linda and I got on well, and I had started Toby on a new and innovative treatment. He was responding well to the medication, which was the same as that used in human patients to treat rheumatoid arthritis.

Sadly, soon after I had sorted out Toby's sore gums, he got hit and killed by a car on the busy road near where the family lived. It wasn't too long before they acquired a poodle called Rosie. Around the same time that Anne and I were having our scans, Linda, beside herself with excitement, brought Rosie in, also to be scanned for pregnancy. With a large grin on her face, she explained how her little poodle had arrived in this situation.

'Well, Julian, we were at Bolton Abbey on a walk a few months ago and we met this lovely couple and they had a lovely little black poodle, a boy, and Rosie and he got on really well. They were such a nice couple – two teachers – and we swapped phone numbers and we said how we desperately wanted a litter from Rosie and they seemed keen and, well, they said next time she's in heat, give us a ring …'

So you can imagine what happened next. When Rosie was next in season, a few months later, a rendezvous was arranged back at Bolton Abbey. Bolton Abbey is a beautiful place, in a sheltered bend in the River Wharfe. It is a great place for a walk on a Sunday and, as it turned out, a great place for two poodles to mate. Just opposite the ruined abbey, on the other side of the river, is a large, flat grassy area, where picnickers and children playing football or paddling in the peat-infused water congregate on a sunny weekend. There is a row of stepping stones to cross the river when the water level is low enough. On this particular Sunday, the picnicking public and their children were treated to a riveting spectacle as Rosie met her lover, Gabriel. Rosie was, apparently, gagging for it and did not even need the comfortable rug that the teachers had thoughtfully provided for the romance.

The couples' own children were dispatched to play in the woods nearby and the adults settled down with their flasks of coffee, to supervise the mating. However, neither Linda, her husband, nor the teachers had experienced this kind of thing before and the humans did not prove to be much help. Luckily, Rosie and Gabriel had a better clue of how to carry on and, oblivious to the large number of onlookers, got down to business. The mating of a male and female canine cannot be, in any way, described as subtle. Once the male has mounted, his penis swells, as if there is a Cox's apple stuck half way down its length. This makes it impossible for him to retreat, as the pelvic muscles of the bitch clamp around this swollen gland. The result is a 'tie', where the two dogs are literally stuck together, at times with their backs to one another. It would have been impossible to disguise the scene. The picnic blanket was hastily held aloft, in the same way as you would when trying to change into your swimming trunks on the beach. It did little to hide the modesty of Rosie and Gabriel (who didn't care anyway).

Three and a half weeks later, as I arranged the scanner and clipped Rosie's tummy to facilitate a clear picture, I tried to warn Linda that the news might not necessarily be good. A mating takes plenty of planning; often pre-mating swabs or blood tests are taken to ensure optimum timing and the environment has to be just right for both bitch and dog. But to everyone's surprise and delight, four pups were clearly visible on the screen. There was as much laughter in my consulting room that afternoon as there had been three and a half weeks earlier, on the serene meadows of Bolton Abbey. Rosie was having babies.

Linda proudly took a printout of the scan and tucked it carefully away in her wallet. I next saw her after the pups had been born. All was well with Rosie, and the puppies were in for their vaccinations and health checks. The story she told about the aftermath of the ultrasound scan made me laugh out loud. After she had left the surgery, euphoric at the prospect of a litter of fluffy little poodles, Linda had stopped off at the supermarket. The car park was pretty full so she parked in the only empty space she could find   in the section reserved for mothers and children. Immediately, a fastidious car park attendant rushed over to check whether she had any children on board. Since she clearly didn't have any in the car, the attendant insisted that she move along to find a different place to park.

'Honestly,' blustered Linda, 'what do I have to do? Do I really have to show you the picture of my pregnancy scan to prove that I can park here?' and with that, she pulled her ultrasound scan printout of one of Rosie's pups from her wallet, and showed it to the car park attendant with a flourish.

'Oh, congratulations! I'm terribly sorry, madam. You are absolutely fine to park here if you're pregnant. And if you would like a hand with your shopping bags afterwards, please give me a shout!'

———

Anne's pregnancy progressed as smoothly as Rosie's and it didn't seem long before we were back at Friarage Hospital, this time not in the dermatology department but in the delivery suite. Once again, I expected it all to be straightforward. Between us, we had experienced thousands of births – lambs, calves, foals, piglets, puppies, kittens, guinea pigs. Admittedly, a human baby's head is somewhat larger in comparison to its body, and to the size of its mother, than that of a calf, but how different could it be?

Ten hours later, Anne was fine and Jack was slimey, but also fine. I, on the other hand, was a wreck. Having witnessed my first human birth, summed up enthusiastically by the midwife as 'Oh, isn't it lovely to have a nice, normal delivery for a change', I could honestly say that I would not have let one of my patients go through that kind of ordeal. I tried to phone our parents to tell them the news, but everyone was out. Desperate to tell someone, I phoned our friend Siân. She was also a vet and due to give birth, also for the first time, five weeks later. 'It was awful,' I blurted out. 'I wouldn't have let a cow go through that.' Tactful!

Having a baby was a life-changing experience, for sure. Of course this was mainly because of the new baby that had arrived, but also because it gave me a completely different view of the levels of pain and discomfort that humans, and in particular women, are capable of enduring.

The following day, Anne and Jack were in the ward for mothers and new babies and everything seemed to be going smoothly. There was a calm atmosphere in there, and Anne and little Jack seemed to be the most relaxed of all. The first few days were going well. By day three, we thought it would be a good idea to give Jack a bath. He was still bloodstained and the gloopy birth fluids were still stuck on his head. I went to find a midwife to organize the plastic portable bath. When the midwife brought over the bath on a trolley, she explained that she would return shortly to show us what to do. 'Fill it up with tepid water, and I will be back in a minute' were her parting words. Some time later she had not returned.

'How hard can it be?' I thought. Bathing a baby is surely just like bathing a dog. Diligently, I set about filling the bath with tepid water. It mustn't be too hot – I'd learnt this at antenatal classes. I was a modern father, and baths and nappies I would take in my stride. Tepid, though? We were both a bit surprised. To both of us, tepid meant just a bit warmer than cold.

I filled up the bath with water and dipped my elbow in to confirm it was not too hot. It was definitely not too hot, it was definitely tepid, but that's what the midwife had said. 'Gosh, how easy this is,' I thought. I grasped Jack, like Simba in *The Lion King*, and plunged him into a bath of cold water. Judging by the noise and scale of his objections, I could tell something wasn't quite right and midwives came running from all directions.

'What are you doing?' exclaimed the now rather cross midwife, who had finally reappeared. 'You can't bath a baby in cold water!'

Eventually Jack calmed down and realized his world was not coming to an icy and premature end, and we were shown the correct technique for baby bathing. The temperature had to be *warm* (and in our defence, the description of the temperature should really have been *lukewarm*, rather than tepid), not cold, and the baby needed to be lowered gently into the water rather than adopting the plunge-pool technique. We, and more particularly I, had a lot to learn about babies. Rearing one, I was discovering, was not quite the same as rearing a puppy or a lamb.

Poor Jack. We really just made it up as we went along, but by the time he was two, we thought we'd cracked it, and just before his third birthday, late and laid back, his little brother, Archie, arrived.

16

Bobby and Harvey the Inflatable Dog

With the arrival of Jack, life at home took a new and different turn. The life of the practice had also changed dramatically in the wake of foot-and-mouth. Farms that had been infected were just beginning to restock after the long cleaning and disinfection period. About a third decided not to return to livestock, and another third returned, but with smaller numbers and less intensive systems, requiring minimal veterinary intervention. The remaining third *did* restock and return to farming in a similar way to before the crisis. These farmers saw the epidemic as a brilliant opportunity to start from scratch and re-engaged with great enthusiasm. This was a very positive time for those of us in the profession who enjoyed a more integrated role as a veterinary surgeon on farms. It was extremely rewarding to be involved from the very first plans, and to have meetings discussing health and management strategies for new systems, what type of animals were suitable and what type of herd would develop. One dairy farmer, after a lot of research, invested heavily in a robotic milking machine. It was the first of its kind in this area and years ahead of its time. Others diversified into different breeds of cattle. Whole herds of beautiful brown South Devons, or shiny, black, pedigree Aberdeen Angus cattle appeared in the place of generic mixed-breed suckler cows, moving the emphasis away from quantity and towards the quality associated with traditional breeds. Apart from anything else, these herds looked very handsome.

The result of these new approaches was that the balance of work at the practice shifted significantly for the first time. Small animals became the dominant part of our working week, accounting for about 65 per cent of our caseload. This was in part due to the relative paucity of farm animals, but also because the pet-owning public was on the increase. Not only that, but there was much more demand from pet owners for more involved treatments, and the success of the television series *Vets in Practice* certainly helped. This series followed a cohort of veterinary students who qualified in 1996, the same year as I did. They were filmed as they progressed through their training and the early part of their careers. It was extremely popular, though I have to say, I was not a regular viewer. Most vets would steer well clear of yet more sick animals after getting home from a busy day. Nonetheless, it was a very well-made programme and it had some great stories and characters. For the second time in a generation the veterinary profession had been given a much-needed shot in the arm by a popular mainstream television series.

The move towards more small animal work provided some brilliant intellectual challenges. Farm work is all about the health of the herd, but with a pet there is the opportunity for in-depth investigations, and specific treatment of the individual. It gives us the chance to delve back into the enormous pot of knowledge we accumulated at vet school, and we can approach cases as a medic or a surgeon rather than a herd advisor.

At around this time, a dog came into the surgery that had the biggest impact on my small animal career so far. His name was Bobby and he was a Border collie. When I first met him he was a five-month-old pup. He was really quite poorly and had been in to see colleagues about three or four times already. On this occasion he was on the list to see me. His owner, Val, was a fairly new client to the practice and neither of us knew at this point that we would be seeing each other, with Bobby, two or three times a week for the next eighteen months and that we would become good friends.

Bobby was suffering from repeated bouts of non-specific illness. He would develop a high temperature, lose his appetite and become listless, but other signs were vague, and on each occasion he appeared to respond to symptomatic treatment. When I first met him he had ulcers in his mouth and was drooling. This sounds just like the disease with which I had been preoccupied for most of the previous year, but Bobby was not a calf nor a sheep so I could exclude foot-and-mouth disease – dogs were not cloven-hooved, I had learnt that ages ago. It is, though, very unusual to see mouth ulcers in a dog, especially a young pup. I arranged to admit him for an anaesthetic so that I could examine his mouth and take biopsies. The results came back quickly but the histology report from the pathologist was almost as vague as Bobby's clinical signs. There were various diseases that could cause ulcerative stomatitis in dogs but they were rare. I took some more samples – this time blood tests – and started cautious treatment. All seemed to go well, so I was disappointed when he became ill again, a couple of weeks later. Another round of blood tests showed a high white cell count. This was an obvious sign of inflammation and probably infection. Despite a battery of x-rays and ultrasound scans, try as I might, I still couldn't identify the cause.

Then the story became even more mysterious. It transpired that Bobby's brother had been treated at another veterinary practice for similar signs. He had been referred to a specialist for investigation of the mystery illness. The specialist, as it turned out, wasn't quite so special, and had failed to get to the bottom of the illness. Bobby's brother had deteriorated and been put to sleep.

The next step, I decided, was to take a bone marrow sample. The bone marrow is the part of the body that makes blood cells – both the red cells that carry oxygen around the body, and the white cells that fight infection, by attacking bacteria and viruses. I was suspicious there was a problem with Bobby's bone marrow, as he seemed prone to infections, so I needed to investigate this possibility. The samples were taken and sent off to the laboratory. The results, when they came back, appeared to be unequivocal – Bobby's bone marrow was alive and well. It was bursting with loads of immature white blood cells, all ready to be sent out to work, to fight infection. The laboratory diagnosis was 'immune mediated neutropaenia'. This meant Bobby's own immune system was actually destroying its own white blood cells, once they had been sent out into the bloodstream, thereby rendering him unable to fight infection. The pathologist seemed confident in this diagnosis, but to me, it didn't make sense. Immune mediated neutropaenia should result in persistently *low* levels of white cells in the circulation and should respond to treatment with steroids. Neither of these things were the case. I phoned the lab. The pathologist, who was an American lady and a world expert on bone marrow, was not in the building, but the receptionist kindly gave me her mobile telephone number, assuring me it was OK to contact her in this manner. She answered the phone straightaway and was more than happy – enthusiastic even – to talk, despite being in the middle of shopping in the supermarket. I was impressed by her commitment. She was very excited about the case because immune mediated neutropaenia was pretty rare. I told her my concerns about her diagnosis, and that I couldn't see how it could be the case. She, on the other hand, was positive about the state of Bobby's bone marrow – the young white cells were bursting to get into the circulation. We agreed to do a further test to see if this was an aberrant result.

After we had done another test, a vague bell started to ring in the back of my mind, about a condition that had briefly been touched upon during our haematology lectures at vet school. I did some research, and it seemed to fit. I thought Bobby might have a very rare genetic disorder called cyclic neutropaenia. It had been documented in a small population of grey and white Border collies. It is often the case that this sort of disorder is carried by a gene linked to an unusual colour. These colours are usually recessive so problems only arise if two individuals carrying the same recessive gene produce offspring. Bobby was black and white rather than grey and white, but all the other signs matched up. The condition was characterized by cyclic variations in the white blood cells in the body, as the cells were released from the bone marrow in waves, rather than continuously. Every three weeks his bone marrow would stop releasing the bacteria-fighting cells into his blood and, in just the same way as happens in a cancer patient whose bone marrow has been zapped by chemotherapy, his blood count would fall. The result would be that his body would be overwhelmed by bacterial infection. This explained his episodic bouts of high temperature. It also explained why, once it fired up again, his bone marrow appeared to be jam-packed with baby white blood cells, waiting to be released.

With Val's consent, and after persuading the lab to carry out the blood tests at a very much reduced rate, we set about trying to confirm the disease, by measuring Bobby's blood count every two or three days, and plotting the results on a graph.

Both Val and Bobby were completely compliant in this exhaustive episode. Bobby simply stood there, or even lay, relaxed, on the floor when I approached him with yet another needle. Amazingly, his tail always wagged and he was always a happy dog, one of those dogs who seemed to wear a smile on his face. He never resented me for being the harbinger of discomfort and, like many dogs I have treated, I am sure he actually realized we were helping him. At times when he was hospitalized with another of his high temperatures, I would sit with him, stroking his head, which undoubtedly ached, but his eyes were full of appreciation. He never once refused to come to the practice and Val described how his tail would always wag and his eyes light up when she said, 'Come on, let's go and see Julian.'

After a couple of months, the graphs we had made demonstrated a clear pattern. Every three weeks, Bobby's neutrophils would plummet to dangerously low levels. Interestingly, I noticed all his other blood cells – red cells, other types of white cell and platelets – also fluctuated, although this did not seem to have the same clinical significance.

So what now, we thought? Bobby was already a year old and had enjoyed a happy life, apart from the few days every month when he felt rubbish. He had outlived his sibling by many months, all of which had been filled with fun. He was on antibiotics and other medications to help his temperature at the times when we expected his white cells to fall, but this was only just keeping things at bay.

I discussed Bobby with the experts, in particular Mike Herrtage at Cambridge Vet School, who was the head of the medicine department when I was a student. He is now a professor and head of the vet school. He was an amazing teacher, and all the students held him in awe. At the same time he was completely approachable, and even well into our veterinary careers he was, and still is, happy to offer advice and guidance if requested. We came up with a plan to try using the recombinant drugs used in human chemotherapy patients, to boost blood counts after toxic doses of anticancer therapy.

I persuaded a hospital to give me some of their part-used vials of a drug used to treat human cancer patients. These opened vials would otherwise have been thrown out. With great caution, I administered these to Bobby, at the times when we predicted his white cells would be low. It worked. The next set of blood tests showed his white cells going through the roof, and we could keep him safe and healthy. Unfortunately, as predicted by Mr Herrtage, these beneficial effects were relatively short-lived and Bobby's condition was not as controlled as we all would have liked.

Whenever he was ill, it was me who treated him. If it was on a weekend my colleagues would phone me, and I would go in to sort out his drip and his anti-inflammatories, and rejig his antibiotic doses to make him feel most comfortable. Sometimes I called to see him at Val's house, in the nearby town of Ripon. It was nice to see him happy in his home environment. There was a track around the garden, where the grass had been worn away by him running, endlessly, with his ball. On my first home visit, Bobby excitedly showed me his ball and his usual route around the garden.

Sadly and inevitably, the episodes of illness got more and more serious, and he didn't respond as well at each occasion. We tried another novel treatment that did ameliorate the fluctuations in his cells to some extent, but during one particularly severe bout, it became evident that the decision to put him to sleep needed to be made. I phoned Val to tell her. She already knew, I think. There is always a certain point at which it is so obviously the right time to do this. It is the point when the eyes suddenly lose their sparkle, and it is always clear to any owner who really knows their dog. People often ask how they will know when it is the right time to put their beloved pet to sleep. It always sounds a bit like folklore when we say 'you will just know' but it's true. When the time is right, there is no doubt.

This was the case with Bobby that particular Monday. Putting an animal to sleep is always a horrible job for us, although we normally know that it is for the best, and we are in the privileged position of being able to prevent the drawn out and terrible suffering that often comes with terminal disease. Although we do this on a regular basis, euthanasia is never a procedure that we get used to, but we have to remain professional, and it is usually this that gets us through, and on to the next thing. However, when it happens to a patient that we have been treating intensively for a long time, when we have invested a lot of emotion, and particularly when we have become great friends, it is a wrenching process. On this occasion it was absolutely awful, and I was terribly upset.

What I didn't know was that Bobby had a successor, also a Border collie and also called 'Bobby'. It turned out that it was a tradition in the family to give all their dogs the same name. Three months later I saw a Border collie called 'Bobby' with the same surname on my waiting room list, and my heart nearly stopped! But this was the new Bobby – the next in a long line. The small black and white and very cute Border collie was just as pleased to see me as his predecessor but, mercifully, was blessed with better health.

There are few cases that are as emotionally charged as Bobby and, in fact, mostly our cases are happy stories, which are uplifting and pleasant to deal with. It is just as well, because we would find it very difficult to come to work each day if that wasn't the case. It is not good to dwell on the negatives, and we are lucky that the pace of our practice is such that it is never very long before a bitch caesarean arrives and we have our hands full of squeaking newborn puppies, or a pair of kittens turn up for their vaccinations, and our faith in the vigour of life is restored.

One of these amusing and uplifting cases involved the dog belonging to Sylvia, one of our receptionists, although I do not think Sylvia found it very funny at the time. Harvey, a robust Border terrier, had been involved in a skirmish with another dog. The offending dog had ventured into Harvey's garden. Being the owner of a Border terrier myself, I knew this was a risky thing to do. Border terriers are very protective of their own patch. Having managed to break up the fight, Sylvia scooped up Harvey and rushed him in to be checked over for battle wounds. The biggest injury appeared to be to his pride, but he did have a number of small lacerations on his throat, which were attended to and patched up by a colleague. This was on a Thursday afternoon, and no one expected anything but a speedy return to normal. However, I saw Harvey as an emergency the very next day. The sight was extraordinary. Harvey's entire body was inflated just like a blow-up toy. Even his head and face were distorted by the air under his skin. This gave him the appearance of wearing a ridiculous grin, because the corners of his mouth were pulled so tight.

Unbeknown to anyone at the time, his trachea, the pipe taking air from his mouth to his lungs, had been damaged in the dogfight, and air was leaking out of it into the loose connective tissue under his skin. I took an x-ray of Harvey to check that there was no leakage of air to other places, as this could have been more serious. While he was asleep for the x-rays, I made various holes in his skin, and air came whistling out, as if he was a leaking inner tube. I also wrapped bandages around his legs, as the air was beginning to seep down there too. If it went all the way to his feet, not only would he look even more ridiculous, he wouldn't be able to walk.

The x-rays confirmed his upper airways were not too badly damaged. I felt confident that the leaks would soon heal over, and that there would be no serious long-term effects. Harvey certainly did not seem in any discomfort. I tried to reassure Sylvia, but she did not seem completely convinced. Her dog looked like Violet Beauregarde, the girl who was inflated in Willy Wonka's Chocolate Factory. I jokingly suggested that she brought Harvey for his next checkup on a string, along with a bunch of balloons, rather than on a lead!

Happily, Harvey did deflate after several days without any further treatment, but his visits during his inflated days were always hilarious, and a perfect antidote to the sad moments of our working day.

17

World Records and Team GB

I have always thrived on pushing myself hard physically, whether during cross country running at school, or rowing, rock climbing and mountaineering at university, or later on my mountain bike. I throw all my energy and enthusiasm into my sports and, for better or worse, I have an overriding competitive determination. I was never content with a 'gentle paddle' while rowing with the college eight, or a 'steady' bike ride with my mates. I always have to be going hard and fast. Up until my early thirties, my greatest success had been when I was seventeen, competing for West Yorkshire, in the English Schools Cross Country Championships. I got my place in the team by a stroke of luck. I was the first reserve, and therefore I didn't expect to get the chance to race. However, the day before the team left for Cornwall, one of the other runners twisted his ankle whilst running round the dark streets of Leeds. I got a phone call at half past nine on the Thursday evening: 'Could you run? We leave in the morning at 5.30 a.m.' I jumped at the chance, and had a fantastic race. I finished nowhere near the front, but just to get there was achievement enough. I trained hard in those days, as I still do, and on that trip to the English Schools, I shared a room with a guy called Mark Sesay. He was an awesome athlete – a junior international – and I quizzed him about his training regimes. As the conversation progressed, I was surprised to find that I actually did a much greater volume of training than he did!

Competition was in my blood. My father had been a national-standard runner, had an Oxford Blue and had competed at the Bislett Games in Oslo in 1963. It was the same stadium where Steve Cram broke the world record for the mile in 1985. My maternal grandfather had been a competitive track cyclist. I was still some way behind their level of sporting success.

But then I was reinvigorated by my change in diet. Looking back I had probably been afflicted by the insidious effects of coeliac disease for many years, which had surely restricted my athletic capabilities. I'm sure that I am not alone in this respect. I am convinced that gluten intolerance is much more common than is generally known. I feel very fortunate that my condition was identified when it was, because otherwise this chapter in both my life and in this book wouldn't exist!

By my mid thirties, I was finally beginning to feel as fit as I ever had. One sunny Saturday, at a wedding reception, I was chatting with a friend, Roger Brown. Anne and I had met Roger and his wife Beccy at antenatal classes, when we were expecting Jack and they were expecting their daughter Lily. Roger is very tall and quietly spoken, but has a fierce competitive streak. He rowed for GB in the Atlanta and the Barcelona Olympics, and has a Commonwealth gold medal. He has competed alongside Redgrave, Pinsent, Cracknell and the Searle brothers and his house is full of pictures of international sporting success. Roger and I were discussing the merits of the Concept 2 rowing machine, used by gym goers and Olympians alike. Roger, obviously, had his own in his garage, and after our conversation it occurred to me that maybe I should get one too. I could exercise to my heart's content on my own rowing machine and, more importantly, I could do it while I was on call. Being on call was, and still is, the enemy of all proper training regimes. If I could row in my own garage, within sight and sound of my pager and mobile phone, I could do as much training as I liked. Going for a bike ride or going for a run was impossible while on duty, and since my on-call duties were every second weekend and two nights a week, it was proving hard to keep my fitness at the level I really wanted. So, soon after that wedding conversation, I acquired my first Concept 2 rowing machine, and I remain convinced that it is the best thing I have ever bought. I could train for an hour a day, even if I was on duty. Sitting for an hour on a rowing machine was the perfect antidote to a stressful day at work. The repetitive rhythm was extremely therapeutic and, as a consequence of this therapy, I became very fit and decided I would compete at the 2008 British Indoor Rowing Championships. I finished in the top ten. I was pleased with my result, but it was so very tough I felt very lucky not to have died. The race was over 2,000 metres, and it was very, very hard. I am not really big or strong enough for the explosive effort needed for sprints. Endurance has always been my forte, and I had another plan.

I had been looking at the records for various long-distance indoor rowing challenges. I did some sums, and reckoned the British record for 100 kilometres was within my reach. The rowing had to be done in a public place, so it could be verified. The gym in Thirsk had just had a major refurbishment, so they agreed to host my attempt as part of their launch. I set about training, and with a huge degree of determination, I managed to break the record, one Saturday in the summer of 2009. It took just over seven hours, and I knocked twenty-nine minutes off the previous record. I had a collection bucket and a sign, to say what I was doing, and to try and raise some money, through my efforts, for the boys' primary school. All the gym-goers gave me fantastic support, and quite a few people popped back several times during the day to see how I was getting on. There was some degree of incredulity at the task I had set myself. One guy commented, 'I didn't think things like this happened in Thirsk.' It was true, but I didn't see why they shouldn't. I was just a normal guy, not an uber-athlete, and I think these things are perfectly possible with dedication, preparation and enthusiasm. I was on duty the following day, and got called to do a caesarean on a cow. I was expecting to be in all sorts of trouble with aches and pains, but found that the only part of me that was giving any discomfort was a blister on my big toe. It had been easier than I expected.

So later that year, I phoned Roger to see if he was interested in joining me for another record attempt. I had my eye on the world record for a twenty-four-hour tandem row. This would involve two people rowing alternately for a whole twenty-four-hour period. We could arrange our time as we wished, as long as we never let the machine stop, and the proportion each of us rowed was broadly equal. The existing record looked breakable, with commitment. Roger had long since hung up his competitive boots, but I felt confident I could persuade him out of retirement. I suggested we could use the challenge not only to get fit again, but to raise money for a local charity. However, my powers of persuasion weren't needed. Without pause, Roger agreed.

We trained hard and planned meticulously, giving ourselves six months to prepare. We discussed hydration and feeding strategies, what time we would start, where to do it and, more importantly, the length of the intervals we would row. We decided to do half-hour sessions and our training was focused on this. Our regime was simple – we just rowed as much as we could. At the peak of our training we were covering 200 kilometres a week. Roger told me that this was more than most international rowers would be undertaking. However, we were going considerably more slowly than they would have been.

The training was fitting in quite well with work. I managed to do a session before and after work most days during the week, and then two or three very long rows every weekend. It wasn't doing much for family life, though. Anne, Jack and Archie (who was four by this time) were very understanding, and luckily had the company of Beccy, Lily and Kitty, Roger's wife and daughters, who were, obviously, going through the same trials. The boys got used to playing around the rowing machine as I toiled away in the garden on sunny days, and Anne was enjoying having a toned and muscular husband, albeit one who needed to eat four kilograms of yoghurt and one kilo of walnuts each week, and who fell asleep every time he sat down. On the evening of my birthday that summer, my training was reaching its peak. We had arranged a babysitter so we could go out for a meal. As we sat on the sofa waiting for her to arrive, we realized we couldn't bear to move. We hadn't had any time just lying in front of the TV for months. While I was training all the time, Anne was having to do pretty much everything else, and we were both exhausted. We paid the babysitter anyway but sent her home and stayed in, on the sofa.

With six weeks to go, I had an anxious email from Roger – we needed a meeting! Two Germans had advanced the world record by a massive distance. Our goal had been increased from just over 300 kilometres to just under 350! The German pair were both amazing athletes and both held their respective world records for rowing a marathon. One was also an elite triathlete and had competed in the Ironman World Championships in Kona, Hawaii. There was little we could do now, though. We couldn't train any more than we already were, and we couldn't really abandon the challenge. The fundraising operation was in full swing, and the Herriot Hospice, for whom we were rowing, were promoting the event with enthusiasm.

And so, the day came. Fuelled by my usual breakfast of gluten-free pancakes, bananas and chocolate spread, we started rowing, again in Thirsk gym, at ten in the morning. Roger wanted to go first, which was fine by me, although it meant I would have to do the anchor leg. I knew this would be the bit where we either met with success or failure, and that thought filled me with some trepidation. Everything progressed according to plan and, as the afternoon wore on, we both felt good. Changeovers were critically important. We had to keep the rowing machine going, and we weren't allowed any help. We had perfected a technique whereby whoever wasn't rowing would unfasten the rower's footstraps. He could then throw himself off the machine to the side, and the other person could leap on to continue rowing. It was quite a sight and the spectators loved it!

As the evening wore into night, and most of our supporters went home, things began to get hard. By two in the morning, we had both hit rock bottom. Roger's meticulous calculations told us that we were still on target, but there was not much room for slacking. A friend of ours, Walter, who was a triathlete and also a sports therapist, came to help ease our aching limbs and sore backs. Lying face down on Walter's massage table with his face through the hole, Roger vomited through the hole and all over Walter's feet. By four in the morning on one of my breaks, I was too weak to stand up and reach a drink from the table. It was only a couple of feet away, but I simply couldn't move. 'This must be what it feels like to be old,' I thought.

It was at this point that Roger began collapsing. He had done this a couple of times during our long training sessions at his house, so I knew it was a possibility. His head would go wobbly and he would drift into semi-consciousness. Each time he finished his thirty-minute session he would fall off the rowing machine, and lie motionless on the floor for what seemed like ages. His rowing pace did not change at all though, and he was pushing himself beyond normal limits. I was hanging on, but could not push myself to that extent. That was clearly the reason why he had been an Olympic oarsman.

As the twenty-four-hour mark approached at ten the next morning, the gym filled with friends and supporters, all there to cheer us through the final push. With seven minutes to spare, we passed the previous record distance, set by the Germans, and I briefly stopped rowing to high five Rog. My sister had asked me beforehand if we would stop once we had broken the record. How little she knew us! I pushed on, with the very last of my energy, to the tune of 'Sit Down' by James. We set a new world record of 364,465 metres (nearly 227 miles). As well as breaking the record, we had also raised £15,000 for the Herriot Hospice Homecare Charity.

It was very emotional for the next few hours. We had both

205

known the record was within our grasp but so many factors could have transpired to thwart us. However, our commitment and determination had seen us through. Who would have thought that I would hold a world record? Certainly not me. Even I didn't think this sort of thing happened in Thirsk! Tearfully, I promised Anne that I would never be so self-obsessed by a physical challenge again. I am not sure Anne believed me, but she appreciated the sentiment.

Our record stood for three years, until it was broken by a couple of much younger Aussies. Unsurprisingly, neither Roger nor I were keen to attempt to regain it. We did it once and that was sufficient, and we do, at least, still hold the record for our age group.

———

I did a few more rowing events with Roger following the world record, but after so many hours churning backwards and forwards in the garage or the gym, I was ready for something new. With running and cycling so strongly in my blood, I had, for some time, thought triathlon could be the sport for me. The problem was that I couldn't even swim one length of a pool in front crawl. My children were both good swimmers, especially Archie, who is currently in the top ten swimmers for his age in the UK. I was the weakest link when it came to swimming. I felt I had set a great example to our boys in my training and achievements on the rowing machine. They were delighted to have a dad who held a world record, and it had shown them that anything was possible, with dedication and hard work. Now I needed to apply this to learning front crawl, if I was to take on triathlon as my next challenge.

I arranged a lesson at Thirsk pool. I couldn't manage a single length. The task of 1,500 metres in a lake seemed impossible. The 40-kilometre bike ride and 10-kilometre run would be straightforward, but getting out of the water alive would be a different matter.

Eventually, with much determination, and help from my friend and unofficial coach, Donna, I could swim more than one length. Archie would accompany me to the pool on a Sunday morning and offer advice. 'Daddy, your feet are too far apart', 'Daddy, your head is too high', 'Daddy, you need to go FASTER!' He was five, and better than me. My first race was an off-road triathlon based around Coniston Water in the Lake District. It wasn't an easy introduction. Most beginners start with short, pool-based races, but I had entered one with a swim of almost two kilometres in a freezing lake, a technical mountain bike course around Grizedale Forest, and a run that went up the Old Man of Coniston. It was a baptism of fire.

I was very nervous before the start, but Donna had briefed me thoroughly, and given me some great advice to make it easier, and give me an edge over my competitors.

'Julian, you must cover yourself in baby oil.' This seemed strange advice, but Donna was a qualified triathlon coach and had competed on an international stage – she knew what she was talking about, so that was what I did. It was supposed to help me slip out of my wetsuit more easily after the swim and before the bike. I liberally basted myself as instructed, and made my way to the race briefing area. I felt conspicuous in my skin-tight wetsuit – it did not leave much to the imagination – but this wasn't what made me stand out. Every other competitor's suit was matt black. I was the only one who was shiny and glistening. By now, despite my fear of the swim, I was desperate for the race to start so I could hide in the water. There must have been an oil slick that endangered ducks behind me as I swam, haphazardly, towards the first buoy.

The water was cold and black, and there were waves, which made it almost impossible to see where you were going. I made it out of the lake about half way up the field, again thankful to be alive. The bike, although tough, brought me back into my comfort zone, and once I was out on the run, I was truly in my element, picking off runner after runner. I ended in a respectable twenty-second place (out of 200 other competitors), unscathed and hungry for more. I could see why triathlons were becoming so popular and I was hooked.

After another season of racing, the old urge to push myself further resurfaced. The ultimate feat of endurance in triathlon, the Ironman, could not be ignored. I discussed it with Anne and the boys. It would mean another prolonged period of life-consuming training. 'Just get on with it,' Anne said. 'You won't be happy until you have done it, and we are used to all the training anyway.' So, in 2013, two years after my first triathlon in Coniston, I found myself on my way to Bolton, for Ironman UK.

Ironman is the daddy of all triathlons. It takes the same format as other triathlons, but over a much longer distance. The swim is 3.2 kilometres (2 miles), followed by 180 kilometres on the bike and finishing with a marathon distance run. Any one of these would make a serious outing on its own, but adding them all together does sound rather stupid. However, as I racked my bike, before the race, in T1 (Transition 1, where we come out of the water, take off our wetsuits, put on our helmets and get on our bikes) beside the long expanse of water that is Pennington Flash, near Bolton, I felt confident. If I finished in the top eight in my age-group category (although forty to forty-five-year-old men is, annoyingly, the most competitive class), I would qualify for the World Championships in Kona, Hawaii. This is the pinnacle for any long-distance triathlete and I knew it was a possibility if everything went according to plan.

Again the swim would be my Achilles heel, and it was, as expected, very hard. My plan was to linger around at the side and near to the back, to avoid being caught in the maelstrom at the start. A mass start of 1,500 swimmers is never fun. It is impossible to see what is going on around you and water splashes everywhere. If you are foolish enough to stop swimming, to readjust your goggles or catch your breath, the people behind simply swim over you, and you are submerged underwater. It is likened to being inside a washing machine and that is a good analogy. A few minutes into the race, which would take me ten and a half hours, I was convinced I would only make it out of the water with the help of a marshal in a kayak. This was because, rather than sticking to my plan of starting off out of danger at the sides, I had noticed a large space in the water, right in the middle and right at the front, just behind the elite athletes (who started 20 metres ahead of the masses, to avoid the scrum). In the excitement of the moment, this was the place I opted to tread water before the hooter went off. As a result, I had a terrible start and was buffeted and dunked repeatedly, as better and stronger swimmers powered over the top of me.

After those first ten minutes though, the race began to go well, and I was soon taking my place on the bike. The course was hilly, which really suited me. It was also cool and damp, in contrast to the searing heat of many Ironman races. Bolton didn't seem quite as exotic as Mexico or Lanzarote, but the grey drizzle had its advantages and, as I sped past my competitors, I knew I was on track for a place at Kona in September later that year.

I whizzed into T2 (the changeover from cycling to running), cheered on by Anne, Jack and Archie, and my mum, dad and sister. It was almost empty of bikes. This meant I was near the front. With blurred vision, I had a quick count up. No more than eighty, I reckoned. Assuming at least thirty of those were elites, it meant I was in the top fifty. As the run was my strongest discipline, I knew it should be possible to hold my position. I swapped my bike for my running shoes and burst out of T2 at great speed. I knew if I ran a three-and-a-half-hour marathon, I would grab a place for Kona. My plan was to run the marathon as four sections, each of about 10 kilometres. I felt fantastic, and ran the first 10 kilometres in forty-two minutes. This was a phenomenal pace. I sped past fellow racers who spurred me on with inspiring comments. One American guy shouted, 'Great running, dude,' as I flew by. At one point I ran alongside Lucy Gossage, the elite triathlete who won the ladies' race. She was a lap ahead of me, but I thought if I could keep up with her, it would cement my chance of qualification for the World Championships. It was a blistering pace, but I figured that the longer I could maintain it, the more time I would have 'in the bag'.

However, the metaphorical bag where I hoped all my spare time was being kept appeared to have a large metaphorical hole in it and by the time I got to my last lap I was completely buggered. Trying to run a marathon at half-marathon pace, it turned out, wasn't the best strategy. I realized I had been racing for ten hours and hadn't stopped for a wee. As I approached one of the many Portaloos dotted around the course I stopped to make use of its facilities. I stood still for the first time in ten hours and stared at the toilet seat. With the door behind me locked, I contemplated sitting down and simply going to sleep. 'No one will notice,' I thought. Thankfully, I snapped out of my reverie, and continued to run, if that was what it could now be called.

When the finishing line approached, I put on a massive sprint (which was completely unhelpful as it happened) and finished in ten hours, thirty-eight minutes. I was seventeenth in my age group and eighty-eighth overall, out of about fifteen hundred starters. It was a very good performance, especially for my first Iron distance race and a good time on a hilly course. Sadly, I was ten minutes too slow for a place at Kona. Archie was cross. As a very competitive athlete himself, he couldn't believe I'd spent all that time in the toilet, and to this day he still thinks his trip to Hawaii didn't happen because of this. I suspect his own time will come soon enough, though. I was cross, too, but it mattered little, since on my last lap of the run I had promised myself never to do this sort of thing again.

That resolution lasted about a week, though, because it turned out that I had secured a place in the GB age group team based on my results in Bolton. The day before the European Middle Distance Championships in Mallorca the following year, I stood on the beach in Paguera and tried to ignore the huge waves and the surfers. The water was so warm that it was to be a non-wetsuit swim. The words 'non-wetsuit swim' make the blood of a weak swimmer run cold. Wetsuits make open water swimming easier because of the extra buoyancy they afford. I had never raced in the sea before and now I had to do so with no buoyancy aid and, unless the weather changed overnight,

I would have to cope with waves that everyone else appeared to be negotiating on surfboards.

Middle-distance triathlons are half the distance of an Ironman race, so the run at the end is only a half marathon. I had reasoned that since the last half of the marathon at Bolton was the bit where the wheels came off, I should excel over this distance. I hadn't factored in waves, but luckily, when race day came (I love the phrase 'race day'), the sea was as flat and calm as a millpond, and the 1.9-kilometre swim was really beautiful. The water was clear and the sun was shining and, for the first time in a triathlon, I could see under the water. Usually it is brown or black, full of pondweed or duck poo, and always cold. This was the opposite and I remember noticing how colourful everybody's tri-suits were, in the national colours of all the European nations. My own tri-suit, at last, bore the words 'NORTON GBR'.

I had a great race, probably the best race I had done, and I was very happy with my position. I was the third GB athlete in my category to finish. As I enjoyed a drink in the bar afterwards, pondering my retirement from competitive racing, a fellow athlete told me that a top three finish entitled me to automatic qualification for the European Championships in Rimini the following year. 'Bother!' I thought, and looked at Anne who rolled her eyes – more training was needed and another six months of juggling the balls of family, work, being on call and training!

18

Things Stuck in Animals and Animals Stuck in Things

No book of the memoirs of a vet should be considered complete without stories of things being stuck in animals. It is a common problem. Dogs and cats have different penchants for the type of inappropriate object they eat, many of which can be very serious but – assuming the foreign body can be removed safely by endoscope or by surgery – can also be amusing.

Dogs have little discretion when it comes to diet, and will happily swallow all manner of inappropriate objects, either deliberately or accidentally. It is hard to understand why a dog would choose to eat something as unappetizing as a mobile phone, but it has happened. Also smelly socks, pants, cuddly toys, cassette tapes, lumps of bone and stones, to name but a few. We frequently have to lever out bits of bone or stick, which have become wedged across the top of a dog's mouth, and one terrier was a regular visitor to have his jaws prized open after they had been glued together by the morning post, which he chewed up as it fell through the letter box.

Dogs have amazing powers of digestion and it is surprising what can go down and be dealt with by the dog's gastrointestinal system, without event. I was once on a farm testing a bull. It was in quarantine and I went to check its health status before it joined the rest of the herd. It took about twenty minutes to persuade the large bull to go into a cattle crush so I could collect the required blood and faecal samples. When I arrived at the farm, the small cocker spaniel belonging to the farmer was busily chewing on a rabbit that it had just caught. By the time I had finished with the bull, the little dog was just finishing the last few morsels of the rabbit, and I could just see its ears disappearing down the dog's throat. Her stomach was bulging alarmingly but the little dog was completely unperturbed, and apart from not needing any tea that night, was none the worse for its bone-laden feast.

One of my patients, a Labrador called Harvey, was one of life's enthusiasts and completely unfussy about what went into his mouth. He was one of those dogs who does things first and thinks about things second. It is a trait common in young Labradors. In fact, I suspected Harvey didn't actually do much thinking at all. The first time I met him at the surgery, as a pup, he had been investigating bees. He had investigated one particular bee a bit too closely and it had retaliated by stinging him on the nose. The result was a very swollen face and eyes so puffy that he could barely see out. His tail continued to wag vigorously and, other than his eyelids being squashed together, he seemed oblivious to his misfortune. The swelling subsided quickly after the appropriate steroid injection but I felt sure I would be seeing Harvey again.

The next time we met, Harvey had been out for his morning

walk around Sowerby Flatts. The Flatts is a lovely area of common land on either side of Cod Beck, the small river that flows through Thirsk on its way to the River Swale. It is a great place to walk dogs, and clients who live nearby often walk across the fields on their way to an appointment at the surgery.

On this Saturday morning, Harvey had spent his walk pouncing on molehills. After several attempts, he had managed to catch a mole before it scuttled underground. He flipped it in the air with his nose, caught it in his jaws and swallowed the mole, whole.

Harvey's owner, Anne, rushed him to the practice. When they arrived there was great urgency in Anne's voice: 'Julian. It's Harvey! He's swallowed a mole. Whole!'

I could tell from Harvey's carefree expression and his continually wagging tail that he was not seriously ill. As I performed my examination, I placed a stethoscope on Harvey's abdomen and listened intently for a while.

'Oh my word! Anne, I can hear him squeaking in there!'

Obviously this wasn't true but I knew I could have a joke with Anne. After a brief moment, during which a look of horror crossed her face, she burst out laughing and all her tension and worry quickly dissipated.

Harvey was fine and after a bottle of laxative to sooth the mole's passage through Harvey's bowels, all was well.

On another occasion, an elderly gentleman shuffled into the waiting room with his Labrador, George (Labradors are over-represented when it comes to swallowing silly things). Through pursed lips he tried to explain what had happened. He thought that the dog had eaten his false teeth. Like all good Labradors in these circumstances, George stood there wagging his tail, oblivious to the gravity of the situation. At this point, it was difficult to work out who had the biggest problem, George or his owner. The old man was sure the teeth were inside his dog. He couldn't find them anywhere. I palpated George's abdomen but couldn't feel anything that felt like a set of teeth. His owner was so certain they were in there, I took an x-ray. There was an area in the intestines that had a suspicious curved shadow, but no obvious teeth. I felt reluctant to operate on George because the x-rays did not show an obstructed pattern, there was no pain and no vomiting (the telltale sign that there is a serious obstruction). Again, it was down to good old laxatives to facilitate a rapid passage. The poor old man was instructed to check the faeces regularly for sign of the plastic teeth making an appearance. He and his dog came in every day for nearly two weeks with plastic bags of poo, so we could check them for teeth. Nothing was to be seen. We even repeated the x-rays, but there was nothing suspicious. We were left to conclude that George had not eaten the teeth after all. I never heard whether they ever did turn up. His owner had to get himself a new set.

Bizarrely, contraceptive pills are another favourite of dogs, and they usually swallow the whole packet, foil and all. The amount of hormone in the tablets is very small, so causes no problem to the dog, but I always feel it must leave the owner extremely compromised. It is tempting, when speaking on the phone to an owner who is at once worried and slightly embarrassed, to try to make the situation better with humour. However, 'Don't worry, at least she won't get pregnant … though you might,' never seems to meet with much hilarity.

I once spent a night removing the majority of a sofa from the stomach and intestines of a Great Dane. The message on the pager that evening said, 'Great Dane. Eaten sofa. Please call.' I didn't believe this could be entirely true, a sofa being a sizable piece of furniture, but by three in the morning, Jon and I had managed to extract about three cushions' worth of fabric and foam from inside the dog. While a sofa is large, so is a Great Dane's intestinal tract!

Cats, for some reason, prefer to swallow long, thin things such as rubber bands, tinsel or cotton thread, with or without the needle. Cats' tongues are very rough, which is perfect for grooming, but something of a design fault when it comes to having a cotton thread in the mouth, because the thread gets stuck on the backwards-pointing spiky bits on the tongue and the only way the cat can dislodge it is to swallow. I remember one cat who swallowed a small piece of cotton thread with a sewing needle attached to it. I immediately admitted the cat for some x-rays of its throat, chest and stomach. Needles and anything metallic show up very clearly on an x-ray, but there was nothing to be seen. I went back to check the story again with the owners, but they were adamant that the needle had gone down. I was confused, so took a second x-ray of the cat's abdomen, this time including the very last part of its intestine as well, although it seemed highly unlikely a needle could have woven its way all the way to the rectum without catastrophic effects. I was amazed to see the needle clearly visible. It was about three centimetres from its anus and had successfully negotiated safe passage all the way through the cat's bowels and had come to a halt just before the final obstacle. I feared that the anus was an obstacle too far so, under anaesthetic, carefully removed the needle with forceps. A normal and safe unaided passage past this point did not seem possible, but it was truly astonishing that there had been no damage at all.

A more unusual foreign body in a cat's stomach was something altogether less spiky. It was a contraceptive, but not the tablet kind. Towards the end of a busy evening surgery, one of our new young vets, Steph, poked her head into the consulting room. 'There's a lady on the phone who thinks her cat has eaten a condom, what shall I do?' I was a bit surprised – it seemed an unlikely thing for a cat to have eaten, but I suggested we see it, just to be safe. Steph admitted the cat when it arrived. Apparently, this condom had been in the waste paper bin, and the cat, who was actually just a five-month-old kitten, had retrieved it. It was, of course, a condom that had nothing whatsoever to do with the owner of the kitten, but everything to do with her flatmate. The plan was to anaesthetise the little cat, so we could have a look down into its stomach with the endoscope. 'Come and give me a shout if you get stuck,' I called into the prep room.

Once I had finished consulting, I went to help. 'How are you getting on?'

'Well, I haven't looked into a cat's stomach before, so I'm not sure whether this is what it's supposed to look like,' Steph replied.

I peered into the eyepiece of the endoscope. 'NOT like that!' was all I could say. All I could see was bright red. It slowly dawned on us that maybe the condom itself was bright red. One of us needed to go and put the question to the young lady, coyly sitting at the very end of the waiting room, ensconced in her mobile phone. Without flinching, Steph went to ask – yes, it was definitely red. Surprisingly, the young lady didn't need to consult her flatmate on this point.

So, out came the endoscopic grabber. This is a fancy piece of equipment, which consists of a tiny pair of pinchers on the end of a long, thin cable. It is fed down a channel on the inside of the endoscope and, by operating levers at the top of the cable, the grabbers can be opened and closed. It sounds as if it should be easy to use these to remove any type of foreign body from an animal, but the mouthparts are very small and, if the object is large or stuck fast, they are often not strong enough to retrieve the offending item. In this case, the offending item was very well lubricated, and it took several attempts to grab it securely. On the first go, all that came out on the grabbers was some unidentified gloop … However, once we got hold of it properly, the whole thing came slithering out very easily. Or rather, we hoped it was the whole thing, as there was a possibility the kitten could have chewed it into several pieces. Someone had to spread it out to make sure it was all there. It seemed obvious that this job should fall to the most junior vet in the practice. For once, it wasn't me.

We see all manner of nasty things in the operating theatre of a veterinary surgery, which regularly cause gasps of 'urgh' and 'yuck', but that particular piece of red latex caused more comment than most, because by now, the story had spread around the practice and any spare vet, nurse and receptionist had come to watch. The kitten was fine, though, and recovered quickly from the operation. We always put any foreign body removed from a patient into a plastic bag and return it to the owner – it seems only polite, if not interesting, and many owners find it amusing. Somehow, in this particular case, it didn't seem an entirely appropriate thing to do.

*

In a world designed for humans, it is not altogether surprising that animals, inquisitive and curious and, in the case of farm animals and horses, also clumsy, end up in all sorts of tangles, stuck in places they shouldn't be. Once stuck, it is often impossible for them to extricate themselves and the vet is usually the first port of call, although in most circumstances the fire brigade would be the more useful emergency service. We don't really have any special skills in rescuing animals wedged in awkward places, but often what is needed is someone to take charge and come up with a plan, and we are generally fairly good at that.

Kittens have a great aptitude for getting their heads stuck in tin cans, while they are inquisitively looking for tasty morsels at the bottom of the tins. The problem is that a tin can is exactly the same size as the head of a young cat, and consequently it is easy for them to get stuck. Again, you do not need a veterinary degree to pull the cat out of the tin, but we are more often than not called upon to intervene in these instances.

Late one evening, a very tiny tabby and white kitten, who we subsequently christened Sticky, was brought to the practice. He looked as if he was only about five weeks old. He was brought in by a chap who worked at a local industrial estate. In keeping with the agricultural heritage of the area, the industrial estates around Thirsk are full of factories making animal-related products – dog food, animal-feed flavourings and additives, ice cream, sausages, cheese flavouring and baby turkeys to name but a few. Some products, if they are destined for export around the world, need veterinary certification, so we spend quite a lot of time in one factory or another, filling in forms. I could imagine, therefore, exactly the place where poor Sticky had been before his rescue that evening by the kind man who was finishing his shift.

The tiny kitten was stuck by all four feet and some of its fluffy body to something called a 'glue trap'. A glue trap is a flat tray, a bit like a cat litter tray, full of very sticky glue. It is designed to catch vermin in an apparently benign way. Once a mouse or rat, or in this case Sticky, stands on the tenacious surface, it cannot move or escape and eventually dies of dehydration and starvation. This seems to me to be unnecessarily cruel and not at all benign. Surely the immediacy of a snapping trap would be preferable. But Sticky had been lucky (in fact, 'Lucky' is usually the name given to kittens who escape a seemingly certain death. In this case though, Sticky seemed more appropriate). Lucky and sticky though he was, he was also in a terrible mess. He was dehydrated, and very thin, but our first job was to free him from his gluey shackles. We clipped fur off his body to extricate him and then set about cutting the glue from his feet. Soon he was free and hungrily tucking into a big bowl of kitten food. He was safe, grateful and quickly on the mend and his condition soon improved. After a night's hospitalization, he was back to full, mischievous health. However, residual bits of glue on his paws had collected fluff from his bedding, so by morning, he had enormous and ridiculous balls of fluff on all four feet, just as if he were wearing slippers. The man who had found him in the trap was more than happy to give Sticky a home, and he went to start life with his new family later that day. Needless to say, the glue traps at the factory were swiftly removed.

'Dizzy', although that wasn't her real name, was another young cat nearly killed by her curiosity. She was rushed into the surgery late one morning. Hearing the receptionist's half of a telephone conversation often gives a good indication of the severity of a situation. The words, 'You'd better bring her straight down!' always sets the pulse racing. On this occasion, the emergency appointment that appeared on the computer said: 'Cat – been stuck in washing machine.'

Before long, a distraught young lady appeared with a cat box and was ushered into the consulting room.

'So, what seems to be the problem?' My usual opening line seemed somewhat unnecessary.

'Oh my God! She's been in the washing machine!' gasped the pale and shaking lady owner. 'I realized too late – she's been in there for over half an hour!'

This sounded serious. She must have clambered into the machine, sniffing socks or looking for a cosy bed, before the washing tablet was added and the door closed.

'Luckily it was only set for a half load, so it didn't fill right up to the top with water, and I managed to stop it before she went through the spin cycle!'

'Too right,' I thought. A little kitten wouldn't have survived spinning at 1200 rpm, and if the drum had filled to the top with water, she would have certainly drowned.

I didn't know what to expect when the kitten emerged from its box. It was an unusual sight. The cat was very wet (having missed the spin cycle, I suppose) and small. All animals are surprisingly small when wet, especially cats. Their normally fluffy fur makes them look much bigger than they really are underneath. Her feet were splayed out as far as possible to achieve a better balance, as her whole head and body went round and round and round, as if she were still in the washing machine. Her face was looking forward and her eyes were trying to focus straight ahead, searching for anything that was stationary. On closer inspection her eyes were going round and round as well. She was obviously very, very dizzy. I listened to her chest with my stethoscope. Thankfully, she had not inhaled any water. This was the main thing, for she could easily have drowned with fluid in her lungs. I could give her an anti-emetic injection that would stop the feeling of nausea and dizziness. We had a new drug that was designed for treating motion sickness, and this was the perfect time to use it. After this injection and by the following morning, Dizzy had made a complete and uneventful recovery and was soon on her way home. On the plus side, her ears were spotless and she was lovely and clean!

Farm animals are no less inquisitive but considerably more clumsy. Sheep have a terrible tendency to get themselves tangled in fences, and lambs often appear to have a death wish when it comes to buckets of water. Young lambs spend the first two or three days of life in a pen with their mother, allowing them to learn to suckle and to form a bond that will keep them safe once turned out into the fields. These 'lambing pens' are usually quite small, so the mothers and babies can form this bond without distractions, and without losing one another, which they are apt to do in a bigger enclosure. However, an unintended consequence is that, occasionally, incompetent lambs find themselves stuck in the water bucket. Dozy mothers are even more of a problem. While on lambing duties, as a veterinary student, I arrived in the shed early one morning to find a ewe that had, unwittingly, rolled over in the night and onto its lamb. The poor lamb was completely stuck between its mother and the side of the pen. At this time we would often refer to sick lambs, which needed extra attention – more milk or the warmth of the Aga in the farmhouse kitchen – as being 'a bit flat'. This particular lamb was, sadly, literally flat. There was no hope for him. Not even the warm Aga would help. He was completely squashed.

When a cow gets stuck in the wrong place, there is often the need not just for the vet but also for heavy lifting equipment. It is not too uncommon to be summoned to a cow that is stuck in a river or a ditch. Their gentle amblings seem to get them into tight spots and their subsequent attempts at freeing themselves often result in them becoming even more stuck.

Late one summer evening, I was telephoned by Alison, our newest assistant vet. She had only been with us a week and it was her first night on duty. I could tell from the tone of her voice that it wasn't the straightforward first night on call that I had enjoyed, twenty years previously. There was no simple sheep with orf or cow with mastitis. She had been asked to see a vomiting cat, but before getting started on this job, another call had come in. There was a cow stuck on a bridge. While this sounded like a line from one of the *Mr Men* books, it was very real, and Alison was worried about what to do. I knew that there would be a large gathering of onlookers, all offering advice: 'Oh, you don't want to do it like that! You want to put the rope there!' and so on. This can be incredibly intimidating for a young vet, so I offered to go and deal with it. I gave her some quick advice about the cat, and left her with that job while I went off to extricate the bovine.

The directions took me into the middle of a large grassy field, from where I could see, as predicted, a growing crowd of people, and some vehicles. The field was uneven, and as I bumped over the grass I was glad of my four-wheel drive. Four-wheel drive is not always necessary for the work that we do around Thirsk, but on occasions such as these, a car with off-road capability becomes essential. I arrived at a narrow footbridge, which crossed a muddy stream feeding into Cod Beck. The bridge was about a metre wide at its concrete base, and had metal railings along the sides for walkers to hold on to. The railings were further apart at the top than at the bottom, giving the bridge a 'V' shape.

There were two policemen, several walkers with their dogs, the local land owner, a handful of youths who had been drinking lager on the grassy river bank, and a fire engine with three firemen hovering nearby, awaiting a plan. One of the firemen was Gary, who I knew well because I had been treating his dog with chemotherapy for its aggressive cancer. I chatted to him about his dog, which, Gary reported, was doing well. This evening's patient, however, was not in quite such a good way. The cow was completely wedged in the middle of the bridge. She looked comfortable and seemed oblivious to her situation, and unperturbed by the spectators. Her feet had slipped off the sides of the narrow walkway, leaving her resting on her chest and udder, jammed between the railings, with her legs dangling down towards the stream below. She was completely stuck and there was no way she could get free without some human intervention.

I could hear various conversations amongst the onlookers about the best way to extricate her. Some spoke of pulling her out forwards, by her head, using a rope. Others speculated the answer was to pull her backwards. Some just didn't know what was to be done, and all eyes turned to the expert.

'F***ing hell!' was the assessment of the situation, from Steve, the plain-speaking local electrician. Steve is a neighbour and friend of mine and I was glad to see him this evening. He works hard and has a thriving business in Thirsk. He and his staff put up the Christmas lights around the town in December and he erects and decorates the tree in the village. He is always ready to help and, crucially, he has a collection of heavy vehicles that can put things in high places and lift heavy objects.

'How the f*** are we gonna get it out?'

'F***ing hell' – again.

'F*** me, we'll have to cut the bars off.'

I managed to stop Steve before he rushed off to get a generator and cutting equipment. I think *his* plan was to cut off the bars and roll the cow sideways into the ditch below, from where he expected she would happily walk away to join her herd-mates. This would not be the case though, in my opinion, as it would result in her becoming stuck in the tenacious mud and weeds at the bottom of the ditch.

'Steve, we'll need your Matbro and some long lorry straps. We'll have to lift her out.'

I had a plan and within minutes Steve returned, trundling slowly but purposefully across the field in his yellow vehicle. I set about shuffling along the bars of the bridge, trying to thread the thick, heavy-duty lorry straps under the cow and to pull them through, so that we could hook the ends onto the long metal forks of Steve's impressive yellow front loader. I clung on with one hand and just about managed to push one end of a strap under the chest of the animal, behind her elbows. I climbed back to the other side and pulled it through. Success.

The second strap wasn't so easy, because it needed to go under her body in front of her udder. Almost her full weight seemed to be concentrated here, and there was no room to push the band through.

Everyone was watching intently now, but the excitement was turning towards despair and there was beginning to be some shaking of heads from the crowd on the grass. She couldn't be lifted by just one strap and so we needed a plan B. They don't teach this at vet school. I asked Steve to get into place with his loader and he could just about extend the front arm so the one strap could hook over its spike. With some straining from the hydraulics, the front part of the cow was lifted slightly – not enough to get her off, but just enough to allow me to push the second strap underneath her body. Once under, I could pull it through and then, with help from the firemen, we managed to heave the second strap backwards so it was somewhere near the right place. Steve lowered the front end of his loader so I could loop the second strap onto his spike and, with gasps from the crowd, the cow started to rise. Had the area been shrouded in mist, the scene would have looked like something from an Arthurian legend. The cow did not seem to register that it was dangling several metres above the ground, and calmly gazed down at the grass and spectators below. Had I been a cow under these circumstances I would like to think I would have expressed some reaction. It must have been the same feeling that I had experienced when I was rescued by helicopter from the tiny shelter on the north-east ridge of the Matterhorn. But this is not the way of a bovine and, judging by the expression on her face as she hovered on high, there was not a great deal of thought going on. She must, at least, have been enjoying the view?

The human element of the crowd (which now comprised not only about thirty people, but forty other cattle, who had come to watch as well) started clapping and there was much excitement. The bovines were not so impressed. One or two sniffed the miscreant, as if to say, 'Are you all right? What were you thinking of? I know, let's go and eat some grass.' And so they did.

It was at this point that the police stepped into action. They tied some special plastic tape across the entrance to the footbridge. I do not think it was to identify the area as a crime scene, but more to deter the cow and its herd-mates from getting stuck a second time. Somehow I didn't think that this was particularly necessary.

19

Changing Times

I recently read an amazing book. I usually read only when I am relaxing on holiday. In the normal course of my life, I do not spend much time relaxing, so I don't read many books. But, during one of our long, rambling but invariably enthusiastic conversations after evening surgery, Tim and I got onto the topic of Laurie Lee, as it was the centenary of his birth. Tim said he would lend me his copy of *Cider with Rosie* and it quickly became one of my favourite books. It describes with skill and beauty the passing of an era after the First World War, in a sleepy Cotswold village. I read it over a weekend in April last year, while I was in Holland competing for Team GB in the European Duathlon Championships. The cameras from Daisybeck Studios had just arrived at the practice to start filming *The Yorkshire Vet*, giving me cause to look upon my life with an outsider's view; but more of that later. Lee's book describes his childhood and the village where he grew up. The character of the village shifts slowly, as motor vehicles take over from horse and cart, and it perfectly captures the passing of an era. It struck me, as I read this book, that the changes documented by Lee in *Cider with Rosie* are, in many ways, similar to changes I have seen, and still see, over my last twenty years as a veterinary surgeon in rural North Yorkshire. Those parallels have become even more marked as I have started compiling my thoughts and recollections for this book.

Nearly all the farms to which I have referred in these pages are no longer rearing livestock. There are many reasons for this. It is not just about the economics, although this has been an important factor. In the post-war period, when it was important to be self-sufficient in food, and when Mr Kellogg was encouraging milk to be consumed at levels never previously seen, farmers were given incentives to abandon the old, low-intensity systems and to adopt new, intensive, highly productive methods. Farming, and particularly dairy farming, boomed. Since then there has been a slow but steady decline in the agricultural industry, and a drift away from the traditional farming way of life. Sons and daughters do not want to commit to working three hundred and sixty-five days of the year on the farm, with little reward. So when elderly farmers get to the age of retirement, the next generation is no longer there to take over. After the two most serious disease crises in memory, the foot-and-mouth outbreak and the BSE epidemic, who can blame them? It is surprising that livestock farming managed to continue at all after these episodes.

Evolution is a slow process, and the changes in Thirsk and its surroundings have been subtle, but steady. This is evident whenever I go into the middle of town. Thirsk is a market town, with a cobbled square accessed by only four roads. This was originally to allow cattle and other livestock to be gathered easily in the square, with only limited options for escape if anything got loose. There is an enormous metal ring attached to the ground in the area where taxis now park. It goes unnoticed by most visitors, but it was used in days gone by to fasten bulls prior to sale.

The days of cattle, sheep, pigs and chickens being sold in the market place are long gone, but not lost from the town altogether. Now the weekly sales are held at the purpose-built auction mart, on the outskirts of Thirsk, where the huge wagons can park, and there is easy access to the main roads. There are still cows, sheep and pigs to sell, and hens, rabbits and all other creatures small and furry or feathered can be seen at the regular 'Fur and Feathers' sales. The evolution of the town and its economy has continued, over the last quarter of a century, probably more rapidly than at any other time in its history. It is easy to overlook this while in the middle of it, but having read Lee's book it has become evident to me that we are in the midst of a period of the most dramatic change in the fabric of rural North Yorkshire.

The decline of farming in the UK has had profound effects on the veterinary industry. The effect most immediately obvious to me, as a senior vet in a rural mixed practice, is the challenge it poses to new veterinary surgeons, starting out in this type of practice. Twenty years ago I would have gone on several farm visits every day, so I could quickly hone my skills, which, once acquired, like riding a bike, would never be lost. Now, with so few farms left, these visits are much less frequent. For young assistants it is like trying to learn to ride a bike but only practising once a week, instead of ten times a day. Without this volume of experience, it is hard for them to become confident. Young veterinary surgeons at Skeldale might get more sleep when on duty than we did twenty years ago, but I am sure every one of the new graduates who come to work with us would swap this for the action-packed nights and weekends of the past. To start a new career in mixed practice now is very challenging, and this is not being helped by the approach taken at many of the vet schools. Teaching is provided by specialists in each field and while this is clearly how it should be, these experts may have had very little experience out in the world of general practice. They are quick to offer opinions on the failings of first opinion veterinary surgeons, while forgetting that if it were not for those of us who see all the normal day-to-day cases, referral centres such as the vet schools would have no custom. One leading equine expert has referred to mixed practitioners as 'Jacks of all trades and masters of none'. This type of attitude is unhelpful and misinformed and does little to inspire the next generation of James Herriots. New graduates are advised to use mixed practice as a stepping-stone to specialization, rather than as a career path in its own right. The result is that there is a poor retention of veterinary surgeons within the profession, so that despite ever-greater numbers being admitted to vet school, there is a shortfall of vets currently in the UK, and particularly in the area of mixed practice.

I spoke with a friend recently, who is a veterinary surgeon. She had visited a small mixed practice high up in the Yorkshire Dales. It could hardly have been more 'Herriot' and Jo said it would have been her ideal job when she was starting her career. This practice had been advertising for a new assistant, unsuccessfully, for over a year. While this is an extreme situation, it gives weight to the concept of the decline of mixed practice.

This should not be the case. I firmly believe that it is perfectly possible to be a good, mixed practice vet, equally able to lamb a ewe, investigate a lame horse, spay a bitch, treat a cat with cystitis, or perform a caesarean on a heifer. You do not need to be a specialist dairy vet to be able to deliver a calf or to pregnancy test the herd. Equally, you do not need to be an orthopaedic supremo to repair the fractured femur of a cat hit by a car, nor an expert in emergency medicine to handle its erratic breathing when you attend to it in the middle of the night. You need to be a good vet, a capable vet and one who works with a passion to treat the patients under your care, but you do not need to be a specialist in every discipline. Sadly, at the current rate, the profession is destined to become top heavy with so-called experts. Generalists, and more particularly good generalists, are becoming increasingly thin on the ground.

I had a case recently that illustrated the point well. We received a phone call one morning from a lady with a sick Border collie called Floss. Floss had eaten a lamb bone, which had become wedged in her oesophagus, below her heart but just above her stomach. The veterinary surgeon who had eventually identified this quickly pronounced that the bone was in a terrible place, and that its removal would require a specialist. The specialist was intending to charge between £2–3,000 for the procedure. This was an impossible amount for Floss's owner – could we do it instead?

'Of course, can you bring her in for ten past eleven?'

I knew it would not be easy. It wasn't easy at all. The irregular-shaped bone was wedged in a difficult place, and the tissues around it were badly damaged. Eventually, and with extreme care, we got it out, and after three days in the hospital, Floss was back home. Ten days later she came in to have her sutures removed, back to full health. It was immensely satisfying for us and we had a great result – a happy and healthy dog and a delighted owner who had saved around £2,000 in fees. As I predicted, it was a tricky procedure, but didn't require an expensive specialist, just an enthusiastic and experienced generalist.

You are a better vet if you are capable of handling all species. Treating all creatures makes for endless variety and no two days in our mixed practice are ever the same. To me it is an obvious career choice. But, sadly, for many mixed practices, the decline in farming has made it neither economically nor practically possible to continue working in this traditional way.

Another nail in the coffin for many small mixed practices in rural England came recently, when the rules for the handling of the statutory testing for tuberculosis in cattle were changed. All cows have to be tested regularly for TB. The test was developed after the Second World War and was an important step at that time, to control the spread of bovine tuberculosis. The drinking of unpasteurized milk was risky if it was affected by the disease. In post-war Britain, the introduction of TB testing was the reason why Donald Sinclair employed Alf Wight and it was the start of their famous relationship.

Until recently, vets would undertake the statutory testing of cattle on the farms for which they provided normal veterinary care, at the instruction of DEFRA (the new name for MAFF). While the work was fairly tedious and often very time-consuming, TB testing was always a good way to get out on farms and catch up with everything that was going on. For practices in the south west, where TB is rife, testing made up a large part of their daily routine. The policy of test and cull has not been a particularly effective one, and the relationship between badgers, cattle and TB has been widely and loudly debated, but DEFRA doggedly carries on testing, and it is a costly business. So, in part for reasons of cost saving, but for other reasons too, the government decided to put the work out to tender – rather than rethink the policy altogether, with advice from scientists, on what advances there had been since 1945. The country was split into 'lots', and each lot was opened up to bids. Our practice fell into the lot that extended from Cheshire to Scotland so it was pretty obvious that individual practices were not expected to tender. A large company won the contract for every area in the UK, and then invited local practices to work under sub-contract. It doesn't take a genius to imagine what came next. We were offered just less than half the amount per cow than was paid previously. And we would have to re-train at our own expense. Decades of experience of TB testing counted for little and we would all need to be assessed to prove our competency. Needless to say, the meeting I attended in York to hear the details of these new proposals was a silent and depressing one. There was no hanging around afterwards for a coffee and gossip or a quick pint in the nearest pub. We used to do that in the past after local vet meetings, but not now.

For us, at Skeldale, it was an easy decision. We declined the derisory offer. We fully expected that this would be the path that most other local mixed practices would take but, surprisingly, most have continued to undertake subcontracted testing at an hourly rate that is about one third of the national minimum wage. The need to accept these terms underlines the financial fragility of many mixed practices and it does not bode well for the future. The compulsion to continue this work is also fuelled by anxiety over the increasingly cut-throat (if not to say unprofessional) competition between farm vets. To have a veterinary surgeon from another practice turn up on a farm to do the TB test could be seen as inviting in the opposition.

When I started my career, each market town had its own vet, treating the animals and farms surrounding it. But as farms disappeared, some veterinary surgeons sought to tempt clients away from neighbouring practices, and a new animosity between vets started to develop in many rural areas. The consequence of the growth and expansion of these 'aggressive' practices has resulted in the veterinary surgeons involved covering huge areas. Rather than being twenty minutes from an emergency, some vets will travel up to 50 miles to see a cow. This is hardly a local service and hardly the best for client care or for animal welfare.

Our biggest beef unit went this way, enticed by the lure of 'specialist' veterinary services. It was the farm where, eighteen years ago, I had spent all day under a leaking gutter, and the same farm around which, later in my career, I would organize my summer schedule of work. They ran one hundred or so very strong bulls that would always need to be castrated some time in the middle of August. We would arrange to do about forty per session. The work was hard and hot and I would measure my exertion by the volume of sweat that I poured out of each of my wellies at the end of the day. One of these sessions had to be cut short when, flagging in the heat, I either lost concentration or the 400-kilogram bull kicked at the wrong moment. The scalpel missed its scrotal target and made a lovely three-inch long incision between my thumb and first finger, laying bare the bones and tendons of my hand. Luckily my suturing skills are good and, with the help of Sarah, our head nurse, I managed to repair the gaping wound.

I was back the next day, with a clumsy and bandaged hand to finish the rest of the job.

It was also the farm where, as a young vet, I would enter the 'calving box of Calcutta'. The concrete-lined room had only one door, through which the cow would put her head and be restrained with a halter, while I delivered her calf. The system worked well until we had to release the cow and get out of the calving box. Once released, the cow would always be standing in front of the door, and we would be between her and her calf. Rather than seeing me as the saviour who had delivered her healthy calf into the world, she would invariably see me as an imposter, and would charge with the full intention of killing anyone in her way. On several occasions in this calving box, I am sure I saw my life flash before my eyes. But then, a new farm management team was brought in, and they were wooed by the marketing department of a self-proclaimed 'excellent' large animal practice on the other side of the county. Another farm was gone.

All this gloom makes it sound as if the future of our practice hangs in the balance, but in fact we are busier than ever. As Thirsk has evolved, so have we. As the farm calls have declined, so the waiting room has filled with dogs and cats, rabbits and guinea pigs, and the day book still has horses, lambs, cows and alpacas enough to keep us at full tilt. That is the joy of mixed practice. More than ever before, pets are integral to family life, and owners expect their animals to receive veterinary care on a par with that offered by the medical profession. This provides us with some fantastic opportunities to push the boundaries of veterinary medicine and provide treatments that James Herriot would never have dreamt possible.

And so, when Leeds-based TV company Daisybeck Studios,

owned by the charismatic and dynamic Paul Stead, approached us in March 2015 with the idea of filming a TV series based around our practice, it gave us pause for thought. We had no marketing department and we had never entered the arena of advertising and promotion. Relying on word of mouth and a good reputation had always served us well. However, the veterinary landscape around us was changing rapidly. A large corporation had bought up a swathe of practices to the north of us, and an American investment company had swallowed up some large practices to the south and east. Simply sitting back and relying on doing what we had always done didn't necessarily seem like the way to secure a solid future. We had been approached in the past by other TV companies – the lure of the old 'Herriot' practice was attractive to the media – but we had never been tempted. None of us really relished the idea of being centre stage, and we felt filming would get in the way of our busy practice. There was also the risk. We had visions of the preview to an episode along the lines of 'A routine operation goes horribly wrong!' or other such disastrous headlines, and we were not prepared to jeopardize our hard-earned reputation.

This time, though, it was a proposition that we felt needed consideration. It could be a fantastic opportunity to champion the cause of mixed practice and promote the surgery, of which we were proud. I felt this more acutely than Peter and Tim who were both closer to retirement than I was. I reasoned that simply standing still was not an option in the ever-changing world of veterinary practice. While we all had strong reservations about the idea of letting the cameras and the whole world into our practice, and it would certainly have been easier not to agree, I had a niggling feeling that if we said no, six months later another veterinary surgery would be enjoying the limelight, and we would be grumbling and cross that we had missed an opportunity.

Peter and I arranged a meeting with Daisybeck, and a lady called Sarah explained their ideas. They envisaged a six-part series, commissioned by Channel 5, to be aired in the autumn of 2015. It would be based around Skeldale, following the day-to-day work of the vets. More importantly, according to Sarah, it would showcase the area, our clients and their animals. Sarah outlined what they had in mind – a 'warm' programme, which would celebrate the beauty of the area and the character of the local people. I quickly realized that we, the vets, would only be one part of the process. This was a relief because although we would obviously feature heavily, there would be more interesting people (our colourful clients), more photogenic subjects (our patients) and the breathtaking scenery of this part of North Yorkshire to distract viewers.

After the meeting, we discussed it at length. Tim was not at all keen, Peter was viewing both sides with equal merit and I was strongly veering towards a definite yes. I reasoned that it would be good for the practice. It would also be a boost for the local community and a real shot in the arm for Thirsk. The Herriot connection has done much for the town. Alf's books and the subsequent television series have brought many visitors and have shaped its identity, but *All Creatures Great and Small* was a long time ago, and today's budding vets have different inspirations. If we were to embrace this programme and if it were to be popular it might help invigorate Thirsk, and bring a new wave of readers to the gentle tales of James Herriot. The worse thing that could happen was that the series would be a flop and we would look stupid, but given the fast pace of the media, I figured that if this were to happen, our errors and embarrassment would quickly be forgotten when the next thing came along.

We didn't have much time to consider our options. Channel 5 was adamant that the programme needed to embrace the truly mixed nature of our work, and in particular, this meant that we would need plenty of sheep lambing. Since our discussions were at an early stage and we were already in March, we had to get a move on, otherwise lambing time would be over. Pete had a week's holiday booked, and I was away for a week when he got back, followed by Tim the week after. As Pete headed out of the practice for his week off, he was very negative about the whole idea. Tim was still a resolute 'no'. I was convinced that we were about to miss a brilliant opportunity. However, while I was away on my holiday in the French Alps, I got an email from Pete. We had to make a decision by the following Monday. I was very excited – Pete had had a change of heart and was back in the 'maybe' camp. Holidays are a great way of getting things into perspective, and he had obviously given it some serious thought. I quickly sent back a very vigorous email: 'YES, let's do it!'

This was followed by panic. What had we agreed to? Everyone had different thoughts on the matter. Some of the staff were very excited, especially our head nurse Sarah who is endlessly positive and always finds the good in every situation. Others were extremely negative and didn't want anything to do with the cameras. This was fair enough, and we resolved that if anybody did not want to be involved, then that was fine. We were plunging into the unknown. Nobody really knew what would happen to our lives over the next six months, but we did know that it would be hard work, challenging, very different and hopefully fun. We were vets, nurses and receptionists, not television personalities, and we didn't know what to expect. Anyway, it was now too late because the following day the cameras were coming …

20

The Yorkshire Vet

And so, the cameras did arrive and we didn't have a clue what to do.

It all happened in quite a rush with plenty of excitement. Once we had agreed to put ourselves on public display, we felt we had to put all our energy into the filming process. If a job was worth doing it was worth doing properly. A couple of days in, I emailed Lou, the series producer, to explain that I had an operation to do on a cow. I thought it would make great television, because it involved two vets, one operating on each side of the animal, to pass the displaced stomach from where it had become trapped on one side of its abdomen to the correct position on the other side, where it would be sutured in place. We needed to head off early, because it was a busy day. As Ruth (the second vet) and I gathered our kit, Lou and her director and camerawoman, Izzy, tried to keep up. I was unaware until later that it was the first time Lou and Izzy had met, as they accompanied me to the farm and watched me strip off to the waist to perform the operation. Lou had set off in the early hours of the morning to drive over from Manchester, and Izzy had found her way from Leeds, having hastily collected a camera with which she wasn't familiar. Still, I reasoned, it was an interesting op and a good one to capture on film. Everything went well with the operation, although it was clear that we all had plenty to learn about being in front of a camera.

Izzy filmed with passion and enthusiasm and Lou watched quietly from a distance, taking it all in. At this point we didn't know that while *we* had made our decision to let the cameras in, Daisybeck Studios hadn't yet made up their minds whether or not they wanted us. They had been looking at various other practices in Yorkshire and, put off by our initial lukewarm response, had cast their net more widely. After this initial insight into the workings of Skeldale, they spent the next few days visiting other practices to assess them for ability and talent. But what we had that the other practices did not have was the fact that all our veterinary surgeons are mixed practitioners. Many mixed practices now have separate departments or vets who concentrate on small animals, cattle and sheep or horses, so while we were neither photogenic nor talented in front of the camera, we could at least all offer a very varied selection of work to the audience. We would literally treat 'all creatures great and small'. Lou realized this and was quick to confirm with Paul, who was in charge of Daisybeck, that her conviction was, in her words, 'Skeldale, Skeldale, Skeldale!'

And so, by the following week, we were back in action. Izzy was swiftly drafted back in, to try and get shots of sheep lambing. Currently we have two camera teams, each of two people working all the time, but at that stage, Izzy was working alone, putting in massive amounts of energy and time. Much of the credit for the success of the series must go to her endless enthusiasm and drive during those early days.

The momentum with which she started the filming was immense and her enthusiasm was infectious. This momentum continued all the way through the next six months. It was frenetic, hectic, tiring and very stressful all at the same time. It was like having to do two jobs at once – our own veterinary job and another one. One with which we were not at all familiar.

One of the first cases I filmed with Izzy was the case of Lothario, the stud alpaca. The practice looks after a couple of herds of alpacas, and it is usually me who deals with them. They are fascinating, gentle creatures, and I have enjoyed gradually building up my knowledge of how to treat them. I had received a call from Jackie, who owned a beautiful herd of these curious animals. They were very well cared for and Jackie was very knowledgable and skilled in their husbandry and welfare. She asked if I could perform a fertility examination on Lothario, who wasn't performing quite as expected. I agreed, with a large amount of trepidation. I had performed fertility tests on countless bulls and rams, but alpacas were altogether more sensitive creatures and I would be in unfamiliar territory. Having a camera crew following me only added to my anxiety. I was still on the steep part of my learning curve with alpacas, and the thought of my morning's work being broadcast on television for the nation's entertainment made it all the more pressured.

I pulled on my wellies and retrieved my microscope from the car. I greeted Jackie as usual, but knowing that every moment of our conversation was being caught on film felt very odd. However, what was to follow was even more peculiar and very amusing. I assembled my equipment and set up the microscope, ready to examine the semen sample I was hoping to collect from Lothario. I had not quite worked out exactly how I was going to do this. In bulls and rams, a lubricated rectal probe is used to provide the necessary stimulation, but this was not appropriate in alpacas and our research had told us that we needed some 'open' females to tempt Lothario into action. Optimistically, Jackie was on standby with a plastic sandwich bag. The plan was tempt Lothario with the female, and then intervene at the correct moment to capture a sample of semen, which I would then analyse.

On 'open' female was marched in to the large pen where the mating was to take place. Head held high and eyes wide open with excitement, she was obviously game, and up for action this morning. Lothario, on the other hand, was very much less enthusiastic. After several half-hearted attempts to mount the female, it became clear that he did not live up to his name. Jackie knew that some alpacas were more selective than others, so a second 'open' female was brought into the pen, closely followed by a third. Some casual flirting continued but, again, no real action. Glancing between Izzy, who was fastidiously capturing all this on film, Laura the associate producer and fluffy boom holder, and Jackie and her helpers, revealed a steadily rising level of mirth. We were barely able to contain our amusement at the ridiculousness of the situation. The final straw was when Jackie decided to introduce another male to the mix, declaring, 'I'll bring in another boy. Sometimes another boy gets things going.'

Izzy was looking expectantly at me to make a comment on the situation. The first thing that popped into my head was, 'This is turning into a proper alpaca orgy.'

We all fell about laughing and the camera stopped rolling as it wobbled around on Izzy's shoulder.

The sampling of Lothario had, on this occasion, been a complete disaster. The morning's work and one of my first introductions to the filming process, on the other hand, had been entertaining and great fun, and much more was to follow.

The case of Monica the ferocious pig was just as funny to film and, since Monica's picture appeared in the *Radio Times*, I am sure this came across on television. Monica is a Mangalitsa, which is an ancient breed of pig from Hungary. Unusually, Mangalitsa pigs are covered in thick, woolly hair. I had been to see her the previous Saturday afternoon when she was farrowing. She had produced three stripy and very cute piglets but Lisa, her owner, had been anxious. Monica was restless and Lisa thought there might be another piglet stuck inside. The sow was aggressively protective of her babies, so it took a very large dose of sedative before I could get close enough to examine her. There were no more piglets inside, and after carrying out as thorough an examination as possible under the circumstances, I gave her two injections to mitigate the risks of metritis, which is an infection of the womb. But three days later, Monica was still not quite right. She could not even be tempted by melons, which apparently were the treat of choice for Hungarian pigs. Izzy and Laura pricked up their ears as I arranged a visit for later that day. Izzy sat next to me in the passenger seat of the car, filming and asking questions. I did not need to exaggerate the possible dangers and challenges of handling this dangerous pig a second time. I didn't want to sedate her again, as she was nursing young piglets, but I wasn't entirely sure how I was going to get near her.

I was soon standing beside Monica's sty. The wall was about four feet high – just the right height to lean on as we peered in and discussed the best way to tackle the job. It also seemed the perfect, safe place from which to inspect the pig who, judging by the noises she was making, remembered me well from three days previously. I could see the perpetual smile on Laura's face slowly disappear as Lisa recounted how one of the pigs had jumped straight over this wall and chased a member of staff right out of the building. Jack, my eldest son, who had come along to watch after school, decided that this was the time to wait in the car.

A plan was hatched for me to inject Monica using an injection lance. This is a device that enables medication to be injected into large and dangerous animals from a safe distance. It is about six feet long and has a loaded syringe at one end and a vet at the other. As I approached the pig it became clear that she had definitely not forgotten what happened last time we met. While she was not hungry for melons, she was most certainly hungry for revenge. I crept into the pen and braced myself for a quick getaway, as soon as my medication had been injected into her woolly neck. Sows look heavy, lumbering and slow but this is all an illusion. Monica's response was lightning quick and she leapt towards me, brandishing her enormous tusks, mouth wide open and saliva spraying. Laura, on the other side of the wall, jumped in the air and I screamed and ran, just managing to close the gate behind me as her tusks clattered against it, missing my leg by a whisker. Safely behind the gate, there was much laughter from everyone, for the second time in a week. I rather hoped that Laura might not have recorded me screaming, in her surprise at the pig's reaction, but as I urged Izzy, 'PLEASE don't put that into the edit,' I knew full well that it would make the cut.

———

People often ask what it is like to have a camera crew following us around all the time. The answer is that to begin with, it was challenging, time-consuming and often intrusive. But over the months, everyone at the practice has become great friends with the team, and we all have complete trust in them, their professionalism and their skill. Without this, we would be very vulnerable. Now we are used to it, we often don't feel as if we are being filmed at all. The camera crew are our close friends, with whom we share the rollercoaster of emotions that are intrinsic to our jobs in the veterinary profession. It isn't a hassle to take them along on a call, or to have them in to film a consultation. It is a privilege to be able to show off our work to anyone who might find it interesting.

It has taken a while for us to reach this point though. Half way through the sunny summer of 2015, my stress levels were at a new high, and Anne and the boys were having to put up with me being tired and grumpy. None of us knew how the programme would be received. We were convinced that we would look silly and inept. We hadn't appreciated the degree of exposure to which we would be subjected and I swore, much like Steve Redgrave after his penultimate Olympic gold, that I would never do this again. I had seen small snippets of footage as they were played back on the cameras, and I had watched a short clip of me calving a cow in the middle of the night, which did look good, but at this point, we had not seen any complete pieces of filming. The first finished piece I saw was filmed by David. He is a skilled and experienced director with a careful eye for detail. He showed me a clip that would go into the first or second episode. It was of me talking on the telephone, to the owner of a cat upon which I had just been operating. It was bad news. I spoke for a few minutes and, unadulterated by background music and the splicing in of cute animal scenes, it was just me blathering on the telephone. I thought it looked terrible and, far from buoying me with excitement as David had hoped, it filled me with dread.

Peter and I had been given permission to view the 'rough cuts' before the final edit and release to Channel 5. This was so we could check them for accuracy. If there was anything that had been portrayed unclearly, or aspects with which we were not completely comfortable, we could say so at this point, and they would be altered. On one Thursday in August, we went round to Paul's office to watch the first episode. We were both very nervous. It was the first time we had seen ourselves as others see us, and it was immeasurably weird. Aside from this, we were both astonished at what had been created from our basic and reasonably inept work in front of the camera. The editors had worked some sort of magic. It was an emotional first episode because it included the story of head nurse Sarah's own dog, Copper, who had to be euthanased due to an inoperable tumour. Sarah bravely allowed this to be filmed and, by this time, knew it would feature in the first episode. We had been adamant from the outset that we would not do things differently just because we were being filmed, and Copper's case was testament to this. Afterwards, when I went back to the practice, Sarah was the first to rush up to ask what it was like. With tears in my eyes, all I could say was, 'It's bloody brilliant!'

Excitement was mounting, both in Thirsk and at Daisybeck. The first Sunday in September was the day the programme would be launched, and Paul had booked the Ritz Cinema in Thirsk to show a preview of the first episode. The cinema is a fabulous place, run by volunteers. It first opened in 1912 and is one of the oldest continuously run cinemas in the country. It has just one screen, with stalls and a balcony, but shows all the latest films, and everyone in Thirsk goes there. It seemed an entirely appropriate venue. The great and the good from Yorkshire were invited, as well as important people from the media world. Even the commissioning editor of Channel 5 had made the journey from London for the occasion.

I had been out on my bike that morning around the beautiful Hambleton Hills, which would feature strongly in the forthcoming episodes. I needed to clear my head and have some time to myself. The fresh air and exertion of a climb up Boltby Bank was perfect. As ever, I had tagged an extra loop onto my ride and was running slightly late. About twenty minutes before the show was due to start, I whizzed through Thirsk market place on my way back home. As I passed the cinema I could barely believe my eyes. There was a red carpet and two life-sized posters each emblazoned with a picture of me with my faithful dog, Emmy. Only a few days before, Daisybeck had pronounced that, since the programme was called *The Yorkshire Vet*, it was important that one of us actually took the title role. That person was, they said, to be me. This hadn't been made clear at the outset but now I was the person on all the pictures and, as I lined up on the red carpet with Anne, Jack, Archie, my parents, my sister Kate, and loads of other friends and colleagues, I sensed that in many ways, life might not be quite the same again.

———————

Six months later, and it turned out that this was a fair prediction.

In many ways, nothing has changed at all. The patients in the waiting room still need to be attended to, anal glands still need to be emptied, cows still need to be calved in the middle of the night. The shopping still needs to be done, the kids ferried to school, hockey, tennis and swimming, and the dog walked. In other ways, much has changed. I knew I had really made the big time when the local fishmonger asked me for a 'selfie', but I was still rather surprised when I was recognized by an airline steward at Leeds Bradford Airport. I was invited to cut the red ribbon to open Easingwold Christmas tree shop, and Pete and I were even asked to switch on the Christmas lights in Thirsk!

It wasn't long before there was talk of a second series. The idea had initially filled me with dread. At one point I resolved to write a note to myself, reminding me of how demanding the filming process had been. The note was to be opened after the first series had been aired as a way of deterring me from doing it all again. But, in the Norton household, we have something of a motto to explain what drives us to challenge ourselves. It goes along the lines of: 'Because it would be easier not to'.

It is the feeling I had when I stood at the bottom of the Frendo Spur above Chamonix, and the feeling I get as I pull on my wetsuit to swim in a cold and pondweed-infested lake. It is difficult at the time and it is undoubtedly easier to turn round and go home, where the sofa is comfy and the glass of wine is tempting. But afterwards, we know that the extra effort will always have been worth it. As Edward Whymper said in his classic book *Scrambles Amongst the Alps*, where he described the first ascent of the Matterhorn: 'The recollections of past pleasures cannot be effaced … there have been joys too great to be described in words …'

He refers to the joys associated with climbing, but his philosophy applies to everything. You rarely achieve these joys by sitting back and taking the easy option.

So with this in mind, we agreed to enter the arena again, and put ourselves through another ten months of potential humiliation and worry. The cameras are back and another series is underway ...

Acknowledgements

While most of the writing of this book has been a solitary process, carried out in the early hours of the morning, the same cannot be said for the stories of which the book is made. Were it not for my workmates, clients and their animals, there would not be a book at all. So my first and biggest thank you must be to my colleagues at Skeldale Veterinary Centre, Thirsk, and in particular to Peter, Tim and, at the beginning, Jim. It has been a great privilege to work here alongside you, and it is a truly unique place to work. Thanks also to Jim for writing the foreword – and for underlining the very special links that still exist between your father and the modern practice in Thirsk today.

Thank you to the clients of this practice, who have been, and continue to be, lovely, honest and genuine. It has been a great pleasure to treat all your pets and farm animals over the years. Special thanks to the Bell family, for their time and the loan of handsome calves, sheep and horses for photo shoots (the lovely South Devon calf on the front of this book is typical of their beautiful stock). Theirs is the first farm in the practice that I ever visited, although it was before I was a vet. While walking the 'Coast to Coast' walk as a sixteen-year-old with a couple of schoolmates, I passed this farm and walked up their drive. Little did I know that, eight years later, I would become intimately involved with the health and welfare of the animals on this farm. Your friendship and, seemingly unswerving, faith in my clinical judgment have been ever present in my time working at Skeldale. Thank you.

Also, were it not for the television series, *The Yorkshire Vet*, writing this book would have been a much more difficult proposition. I am very grateful to Paul Stead of Daisybeck Studios in Leeds, for approaching us in the spring of 2015 and for his faith in our ability to hold together not one but three series of programmes. Your encouragement, commitment and fervour have been brilliant. Moreover, the team of directors, producers and editors has been a joy to work with. When being filmed we are completely at your mercy and we are all extremely grateful for your sympathetic treatment! Producer directors Izzy Arrieta, David Terry and especially Laura Blair, I'll never forget the funny, emotional and sometimes smelly moments we have enjoyed together. Series producer, Lou Cowmeadow, thank you for being so great and looking after us all. Also, enormous thanks to Natasha Jarvis, associate producer in series two, for your unflagging enthusiasm and also for your brilliant photos featured here on the front and back cover.

Thanks go to the staff at Michael O'Mara Books, particularly my editor, Louise Dixon, and publicist, Clara Nelson for so positively engaging with this book; you have both been a great help and made this first effort such fun. Another person without whom there would be no book is my agent, David Riding, from MBA Literary Agents, who spotted the potential after the first episode of series one. Thank you for your vision!

My heartfelt thanks must go to my family: my parents and sister for their perennial support, despite their increasing incredulity at my situation, but more particularly to Anne and our boys, Jack and Archie. Despite many hours away from home – on call, training and, more recently, writing, I have never heard a single complaint from any of you and I am so grateful – thank you.

Finally, to Anne, thank you for putting up with my occasional grumpy tempers – and all my other faults – and also for expertly editing this text. Mine was the easy bit because the stories were in my head, but knocking them into readable sense was the hard bit. Without you, both this book and my life in general would be considerably less good!